Essentials of Pharmacology
for Nurses

Essentials of Pharmacology for Nurses

Paul Barber and Deborah Robertson

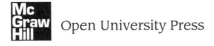

Open University Press
McGraw-Hill Education
McGraw-Hill House
Shoppenhangers Road
Maidenhead
Berkshire
England
SL6 2QL

email: enquiries@openup.co.uk
world wide web: www.openup.co.uk

and Two Penn Plaza, New York, NY 10121-2289, USA

First published 2009
Reprinted 2009 (twice), 2010, 2011
First published in this second edition 2012

A catalogue record of this book is available from the British Library

ISBN-13: 9780335245659 (pb)
ISBN-10: 033524565X (pb)
e-ISBN: 9780335245666

Library of Congress Cataloging-in-Publication Data
CIP data has been applied for

Typeset by Aptara Inc., India
Printed and bound by CPI Group (UK) Ltd, Croydon, CR0 4YY

Fictitious names of companies, products, people, characters and/or data that may be used herein (in case studies or in examples) are not intended to represent any real individual, company, product or event.

The McGraw·Hill Companies

Praise for this book

"This book is excellent in terms of how it explains complex ideas into simplified terms … It's a practical guide to drugs used in nursing, telling you drug types, effects on the body and side effects the client might encounter. This piece proves to be an excellent piece of kit for nurses from all specialties! A truly invaluable book for students and nurses alike."

Carol Molly Casey, University of Wolverhampton (RnDipHE), UK

"This key book is an essential purchase for all current and forthcoming nursing students … It is easy to read, clearly written and follows a logical path through a wide scope of subjects relating to pharmacology in nursing … This book will enable the student reader to develop the necessary knowledge and understanding to be a competent, safe and caring nurse."

Keith Booles, Senior Nurse Lecturer/Module Leader, Adult Nursing Practice, Faculty of Health, Staffordshire University, UK

"This book is easy to read with clear explanations throughout and suitable for all branches of nurse education. Each chapter has clear learning objectives, clinical tips to aid thinking and supported with case studies and multiple choice questions … There are clear links to clinical practice throughout. I would recommend this as a core book to all nursing students undertaking nurse education."

Lesley Drayton, Senior Lecturer, Anglia Ruskin University, UK

"This second edition … provides excellent case studies that [make the subject] come alive by engaging with and applying the theory to realistic patient scenarios along with the very practical 'clinical tips'. This is an excellent introductory text both for pre-registration nurses to prepare them for them today's modern nursing roles and also for those post registration nurses embarking on prescribing courses … The format is easy to read and breaks down barriers encouraging the reader to delve into this exciting subject."

Karen Ford, Programme leader for Non-Medical Prescribing, De Montfort University, UK

Contents

About the authors   xi
List of abbreviations   xiii

Introduction   1

1. Pharmacodynamics and pharmacokinetics   **3**
      Learning objectives   3
      Introduction   4
      Absorption   4
      Distribution   6
      Biotransformation   6
      Excretion   7
      General and molecular aspects   8
      Drug action   8
      Agonistic and antagonistic drug action   9
      Drug specificity   10
      Basic introduction to units and conversions   10
      Case studies   12
      Key learning points   12
      Calculations   14
      Multiple choice questions   15
      Recommended further reading   16

2. Adverse drug reactions and interactions   **17**
      Learning objectives   17
      Introduction   18
      Main mechanisms of drug interactions   18
      Adverse drug reactions   19
      Clinical significance of drug interactions to the patient   20
      Major groups of drugs involved in adverse drug reactions   21
      Steps in minimizing the effects of adverse drug reactions   21
      Age-related adverse drug reactions   22
      Case studies   24
      Key learning points   24
      Multiple choice questions   26
      Recommended further reading   27

3. Local anaesthetics and analgesics   **29**
      Learning objectives   29
      Introduction   30
      Types of pain   34
      Local anaesthetics   36

The analgesic ladder 39
Non-steroidal anti-inflammatory drugs 40
Paracetamol 42
Opioid analgesics 43
Opioid antagonists 46
Case studies 46
Key learning points 47
Calculations 48
Multiple choice questions 49
Recommended further reading 51

4. Antimicrobials **53**
Learning objectives 54
Introduction 54
Interference with folate 55
Beta-lactam antibiotics 56
Interference with protein synthesis 58
Inhibition of bacterial DNA 60
Antibiotic resistance 61
Issues with neonates and children 61
Drugs used to treat tuberculosis 62
Viral disease 63
Human immunodeficiency virus 64
Other antiviral drugs 66
Fungal infections 68
Antifungal drugs 69
Protozoa 72
Case studies 75
Key learning points 75
Calculations 78
Multiple choice questions 79
Recommended further reading 80

5. Anti-inflammatory drugs **83**
Learning objectives 83
Introduction 84
Non-steroidal anti-inflammatory drugs 86
Cyclo-oxygenase pathway 2 inhibitors 88
Aspirin 88
Paracetamol 89
Histamine 89
Steroids 89
Antirheumatoid drugs 91
Case studies 94
Key learning points 94
Calculations 97
Multiple choice questions 97
Recommended further reading 99

6. Anticoagulant therapy   **101**

Learning objectives   101
Introduction   102
Blood clotting and the development of thrombosis   103
Drugs that act on the clotting cascade   104
Case study   109
Key learning points   110
Calculations   112
Multiple choice questions   112
Recommended further reading   114

7. Drugs used in chronic conditions   **115**

Learning objectives   116
Introduction   116
Asthma   116
Drugs used in treating asthma   118
Chronic obstructive pulmonary disease   121
Diabetes   122
Medicine management of diabetes   123
Hypertension   128
Parkinson's disease   132
Epilepsy   135
Case studies   139
Key learning points   140
Calculations   142
Multiple choice questions   142
Recommended further reading   144

8. Drugs used in mental health   **147**

Learning objectives   147
Introduction   148
Anxiety   148
Medicine management of anxiety   149
Depression   152
Medicine management of depression   153
Psychosis   157
Case studies   160
Key learning points   161
Calculations   163
Multiple choice questions   163
Recommended further reading   165

9. Patient concordance   **167**

Learning objectives   167
Introduction   168
Adherence, compliance and concordance   168
Factors influencing effective medicine use and concordance   169
Patient empowerment in chronic disease management   171

Case studies 173
Key learning points 173
Calculations 174
Multiple choice questions 175
Recommended further reading 177

10.   Legal and professional issues   **179**
Learning objectives 179
Introduction 180
The correct patient 180
The correct medicine 180
The correct dose 181
The correct site and method of administration 182
Covert administration of medicines 182
Mental capacity and competence in consent 183
Alteration of medicines 184
Reporting of drug errors 184
Controlled drugs 185
Supply and administration of medicines 186
Prescribing law and non-medical prescribing 186
Case studies 188
Key learning points 188
Multiple choice questions 190
Recommended further reading 192

Conclusion 193
Glossary 195
Answers 197
Index 205

About the authors

Paul Barber

Paul Barber (MSc Practitioner Research, BSc (Hons) Nursing, Dip N (Lond), Cert Ed, RNT, SRN, RMN) commenced his nursing career in 1974 as a cadet nurse, where he completed both his Registered Mental Nurse and State Registered Nurse training. Paul spent his early career in surgery, high dependency and accident and emergency and then progressed to become manager of a small surgical unit. Paul commenced a teaching career in October 1988 and has held a variety of positions in education from senior lecturer to head of an educational centre. Paul's current role is that of senior lecturer and he teaches both pre- and post-registration nurses.

Dr Deborah Robertson

Debbie Robertson joined the faculty of Health and Social Care at University of Chester in 2004, where she is currently employed as a senior lecturer. Debbie is an RGN but also holds a BSc (Hons) and PhD in Pharmacology. She is programme leader for the Non-Medical Prescribing Course where she uses her expertise in pharmacology. Debbie also contributes to other modules within the faculty including Research in Clinical Practice, Contemporary Aspects of Healthcare Provision and inputs into the pre-registration nursing curriculum. Her publications to date are derived from her time as a research scientist where she investigated the effects of stress in depression. Her current research interests involve e-learning and the delivery of the Non-Medical Prescribing course.

List of abbreviations

ACE	angiotensin-converting enzyme	MHRA	Medicines & Healthcare Products Regulatory Agency
ADE	adverse drug event	NARI	noradrenaline reuptake inhibitor
ADR	adverse drug reaction	NG	nasogastric
AIDS	acquired immuno-deficiency syndrome	NICE	National Institute for Health and Clinical Excellence
BBB	blood-brain barrier	NIDDM	non-insulin dependent diabetes mellitus
BNF	British National Formulary		
CMP	clinical management plan	NMC	Nursing and Midwifery Council
COAD	chronic obstructive airways disease	NPSA	National Patient Safety Agency
COPD	chronic obstructive pulmonary disease	NRM	nucleus raphe magnus
CR	controlled release	NSAID	non-steroidal anti-inflammatory drug
CSF	cerebrospinal fluid	OCD	obsessive-compulsive disorder
CSM	Committee on Safety of Medicines	PABA	para-amino benzoate/ para-aminobenzioc acid
CTZ	chemoreceptor trigger zone		
DMARD	disease-modifying antirheumatoid drug	PAG	periaqueductal grey
DNA	deoxyribonucleic acid	PEG	percutaneous endoscopic gastrostomy
EPSE	extra-pyramidal side-effect	PGD	Patient Group Direction
GABA	gamma-aminobutyric acid	OTC	over the counter
GABA-A	GABA receptor sub type A	PTSD	post-traumatic stress disorder
GI	gastrointestinal	RNA	ribonucleic acid
GTN	glyceryl trinitrate	SC	subcutaneous
HIV	human immunodeficiency virus	SSRI	selective serotonin re-uptake inhibitor
IDDM	insulin-dependent diabetes mellitus	STD	sexually transmitted disease
IM	intramuscular	TB	tuberculosis
INR	international normalized ratio	TCA	tricyclic antidepressant
IV	intravenous	VTE	venous thromboembolism
MAOI	monoamine oxidase inhibitor	WHO	World Health Organization
MDI	metered dose inhaler		

Introduction

As this book is primarily for undergraduate nursing students it seems fitting that we let them begin the introduction.

'Nurses need pharmacology education so they can inform the patient of what they're giving, why they're giving it and what its going to do to them, and what to look out for.'

'The patient needs to know what they're taking, why they're taking it and when to take it, they need to know what it's for precisely, and its precise function in their life so that they take it seriously.'

'Pharmacology education will be important in the future because the nurse's role is expanding, taking more away from junior doctors. Nurse prescribing is expanding in the community, and is probably going to happen more in hospitals.'

'I think I had about two separate sessions that lasted about an hour. It was definitely not enough, we complained about it several times actually, that we should have had more pharmacology sessions. I'm sure they could have fitted a few more pharmacology sessions in.'

Where then do we start with the process of education? It is our belief that the key to education is through a process of motivation. We both remember, as students, sitting and trying to come to terms with scientific language and almost falling asleep in an attempt to unravel the intricacies of mathematical formulae and biochemical presentations of molecular function.

Learning about medicines is a fundamental part of the nurse's role, whichever field of nursing you decide to choose as a career pathway. This book is written in an attempt to bring to life and engage you in the subjects of pharmacology and calculation of drugs. First, you will notice that not all drugs

are listed. Indeed, we have tried to focus on some of the major drug groups so as to give you a taste of how interesting the subject can be, without initially overwhelming you. Each of the chapters that discusses major drug groups has been enhanced by the inclusion of relevant aspects of physiology.

When putting the initial idea for the book together, we decided that it should include both aspects of pharmacology and drug calculations. However, the book does not contain detailed types of formulae – rather it gives you a basic structure on which to build. We wanted the calculations to reflect each of the chapter's contents and give you a sense of what might be expected in practice. You will not find many examples of the giving of intravenous fluids, because we felt this to be well covered in other texts, some of which you will find in the recommended reading section at the end of each chapter. These sections deliberately repeat the key texts in this field for your ease of reference, and in addition include works specific to the chapter's topic.

A further feature of the book is the inclusion of case studies. Most chapters contain at least two scenarios and, unlike most other books, we have included examples of some of the points that you should have been considering in analysing each case.

Where possible we have also tried to focus the pharmacology on nursing practice. You will notice that in each chapter there are several boxes entitled 'Clinical tip'. These are designed to increase your understanding of the importance of pharmacology within nursing. They should also assist you in reflecting on your everyday practice in medicines' management.

Finally, we have included 10 multiple choice questions for each of the 10 chapters in the book. All the questions are based on information included in the chapter so there are no trick questions. We thought the idea of evaluating what you have gained in knowledge from reading each chapter was important and we hope you enjoy getting them all right!

Well dear student, it is now time to embark on what we hope will be a fascinating journey. We hope this journey will assist you with your initial learning needs, inspire you to ask more questions, and also motivate you to move on to more detailed texts. As we said earlier, motivation is the key to education. You are now our judge and jury. Enjoy!

Pharmacodynamics and pharmacokinetics

1

Chapter contents

Learning objectives
Introduction
Absorption
Distribution
Biotransformation
 Hepatic metabolism
Excretion
General and molecular aspects
 Receptors
 Ion channels
 Enzymes
 Transport systems

Drug action
 First pass metabolism
 The concept of affinity
Agonistic and antagonistic drug action
Drug specificity
Basic introduction to units and conversions
 Basic formula
Case studies
Key learning points
Calculations
Multiple choice questions
Recommended further reading

Learning objectives

After studying this chapter you should be able to:

- Understand what is meant by pharmacokinetics and pharmacodynamics.
- Describe aspects of absorption, distribution, metabolism and excretion of a drug.
- List the principal routes of drug administration.
- Name the phases in hepatic metabolism.
- Describe what is meant by the term 'cell receptor'.
- Understand the concept of receptor occupancy.
- Outline how drugs affect the body.
- Give three examples of different cell receptors.
- Outline what is meant by 'ion channel'.
- Describe the term 'first pass metabolism'.
- Understand at a basic level the term 'affinity'.
- Differentiate between a drug that is an agonist and a drug that is an antagonist.
- Use basic maths to calculate simple drug dosages.

Introduction

Part of the nurse's role, alongside the pharmacist, is the need to ensure that medicines are administered appropriately. That is why it is essential that the nurse has a good knowledge and understanding of pharmacology and the relevant calculations in terms of patient care. Pharmacology is the study of drugs (chemicals) and their interactions with the body. The term is derived from the Greek *pharmakon* which can mean both 'remedy' and 'poison'. In modern medical practice we use drugs more and more to treat and manage disease, so it is vital that nurses understand the basic mechanisms of drug action and reaction.

The aim of this chapter is to introduce the basic principles of pharmacology in relation to nursing practice. The chapter will give you an appreciation of *pharmacodynamics* and *pharmacokinetics*. It will identify the main targets for drug action and allow you to develop an understanding of drug absorption, distribution, metabolism and excretion.

Put simply:

- *pharmacodynamics* is the effect that drugs have on the body; while
- *pharmacokinetics* is the study of the way in which drugs move through the body during absorption, distribution, metabolism and excretion.

For drugs to produce their effects they must interact with the body. This can happen in many ways and depends on the properties of the drug, and will be discussed later in this chapter. Pharmacokinetics influences decisions over the route of administration. The processes that occur after drug administration can be broken down into four distinct areas (known as ADME):

A Absorption of the drug
D Distribution of the drug molecules
M Metabolism of the parent drug
E Excretion or elimination of the drug and its metabolites

Absorption

Before a drug can begin to exert any effect on the body it has to be absorbed into the body systems. This absorption process can be affected by many things but the main factor relating to absorption is the route of administration (see Box 1.1).

It is important that nurses understand the implications attached to choosing routes of administration of drugs based on their absorption. Many patients may need to have their medication administration tailored to their particular medical condition or the medication which they are prescribed, and this is an important factor to consider as it can impact on the patient's ability or desire to take their medication.

Other factors controlling the rate and reliability of drug absorption can be said to be *physiological* or *physico-chemical*.

Physiological factors relate to human physiological functions:

- **Blood flow to absorbing site.** The better the blood supply to the area the greater the rate of absorption. Therefore if a person has a good circulation they will have the ability to absorb the drug well.
- **Total surface area for absorption.** The greater the surface area the greater the rate of absorption. The intestine has a very large surface area, making it an ideal target for drug absorption. This is why you will find that most drugs are given orally where possible.
- **Time of arrival and contact time at absorption site.** The longer the drug is in contact with the absorbing surface the greater the rate of absorption. This is why if a person is suffering from diarrhoea the chances of a drug given orally being absorbed completely are lowered and other means of administration must be considered.

Physico-chemical factors relate to the chemical make-up of the drug in relation to human physiological function:

Box 1.1 Principal routes of drug administration

ROUTE	ADVANTAGES	DISADVANTAGES
ENTERAL ROUTES		
ORAL	Convenient, non-sterile, good absorption for most drugs	Gastrointestinal (GI) irritation, potential for interactions, first pass destruction, inactivated by acids, variable absorption
SUBLINGUAL/BUCCAL	Avoids first pass (see p. 9), avoids gastric acid	Few preparations suitable
RECTAL	Avoids first pass, avoids gastric acid	Less dignified for the patient
PARENTERAL (refers to IV, IM and SC) ROUTES		
INTRAVENOUS (IV)	Rapid action, complete availability	Increased drug levels to heart, must be sterile, risk of sepsis and embolism
INTRAMUSCULAR (IM)	Rapid absorption	Painful, risk of tissue damage
SUBCUTANEOUS (SC)	Good for slower absorption	Absorption variable
INHALED (LUNGS)	Large absorption area, good for topical use	Few disadvantages

Other routes include intra-arterial, intrasternal, intrathecal, intra-articular, intraperitoneal, intraventricular, nasal, bronchial, vaginal, skin and conjunctiva

- **Solubility.** How soluble is the drug in body fluids? As the body is made up of a large amount of water, drugs can dissolve readily. However, certain drugs do not dissolve into small enough particles to ensure rapid absorption.
- **Chemical stability.** Will it break down readily?
- **Lipid to water partition coefficient.** Is it more fat soluble than water soluble? This is an important area to consider. As your cells are made up of a phospho-lipid layer, any drug that can dissolve well in lipids will pass through your tissues far more rapidly. Examples of drugs that are highly lipid soluble are anaesthetic agents and benzodiazepines.
- **Degree of ionization.** Some drugs are weak acids and weak bases (alkalis). These drugs tend to disassociate when given to a person.

This means that some of the drug remains active and some is inactive. Often this depends on the pH of the solution (i.e. its acidity or alkalinity) in which the drug is being dissolved. For example, a weak acid does not disassociate as much if dissolved in an acid environment. This means that the drug can cross membranes in a more active form than if it had been dissolved in a neutral or base solution.

Distribution

Once drugs have been administered and absorbed, they have to be distributed to their site of action. For some drugs that site is known and such drugs are available to give locally or topically. All other drugs need to be distributed throughout the body.

There are four main elements to this:

1. **Distribution into body fluids.** These are mainly plasma, interstitial fluid and intracellular fluid. Molecular targets for drugs are found in these areas.

2. **Uptake into body tissues/organs.** Specific tissues take up some drugs – for example, iodine and thyroid gland.

3. **Extent of plasma protein binding.** Plasma proteins such as albumin can bind drug molecules. This varies widely among drugs. Drugs bound to plasma proteins are pharmacologically inert; only free drugs are active. Some drugs do not bind (e.g. caffeine) and some are highly bound (e.g. warfarin which is 99 per cent bound to plasma proteins). Some drugs can displace others from their binding sites on the plasma proteins – for example, phenylbutazone can displace warfarin from plasma proteins. This is an important consideration for drugs which have this effect.

4. **Passage through barriers.** The two main examples are the placenta and the blood-brain barrier (BBB). Drugs must be highly lipid soluble to pass across these barriers. If not, they may not be able to reach their site of action.

The factors which affect drug distribution are taken into consideration by drug companies when developing and formulating medications. While these factors are of interest, the nurse's role in monitoring drug distribution is mainly in monitoring the onset of the effect of, or the response to, the medication. If analgesia is given and the patient reports reduced or relieved pain, the drug has been distributed to its target site.

Biotransformation

Biotransformation of drugs is the process of metabolizing the parent drug compound and occurs mainly in the liver (hence the term *hepatic metabolism*) to different compounds called metabolites. The drug metabolite may have decreased, increased or undergone no change in pharmacological activity compared to the parent drug. It may also have a different activity. Some drugs are what are termed *pro-drugs* – that is the drug itself is pharmacologically inactive until it is metabolized by the liver to its active form. A good example is codeine, which is metabolized to morphine by the body. The metabolite is more

Phase	Process
Phase I metabolism	Oxidation
	Reduction
	Hydrolysis
Phase II metabolism	Conjugation

Table 1.1 Metabolic phases and processes

polar (i.e. chemically charged) than the parent drug and therefore is more readily excreted by the kidney. Drug metabolism can influence dose and frequency of dosing. Drugs which are metabolized quickly have a short duration of action and need to be administered more often (two, three or four times daily). Drugs which are metabolized slowly can have a longer duration of action and may only need to be given on a once-daily basis.

Hepatic metabolism
The terms shown in Table 1.1 are different chemical reactions that change the properties of drugs to facilitate their removal from the body by excretion. Most drugs undergo phase I oxidation followed by phase II conjugation.

Clinical tip

It is important as a nurse to recognize that babies, particularly those less than 6 months old may not have a mature liver and therefore drugs are given with great caution.
Also, patients who have diseases which have an impact on liver function – for example, congestive heart failure, should be given drugs cautiously as their ability to metabolize a given drug will be greatly impaired.

Excretion
Once drugs have had their desired effect they need to be excreted by the body. Principles of excretion include renal elimination and clearance, secretion into bile for faecal elimination and entero-

hepatic recirculation. As previously outlined, some drug metabolites can also have pharmacological effects. If these compounds were not eliminated, they would accumulate in the bloodstream and could cause toxic and unwanted effects.

The main method of renal elimination is by active glomerular filtration. This is where ionized drugs are actively secreted into the proximal tubule. These ionized compounds are actively excreted by the kidney and are 'pushed' out into urine. A more passive form of drug compound movement occurs in the distal tubule of the kidney. Here there is passive reabsorption and excretion of drug molecules and metabolites according to a concentration gradient. Molecules move from a high concentration to a lower concentration by diffusion. This applies to unionized compounds (drugs without charge), and prevents the entire dose of a drug being excreted at once. This helps to maintain circulating plasma levels to allow the drug effect to continue until the next dose is taken.

Clinical tip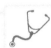

People who have renal impairment may require dosage alterations to achieve a therapeutic level. Older patients also need special consideration, as the kidney does not perform as well as we get older, resulting in a lower glomerular filtration rate.

Excretion into bile is another method of eliminating drug molecules and metabolites. These are secreted from the liver into bile and into the gut for faecal elimination. As in renal excretion, not all of the drug and its metabolites are eliminated entirely at once. Some drugs undergo enterohepatic recirculation. This is where some of the drug is reabsorbed from the gut, back into the bloodstream and represented to the liver for further metabolism. This can help to maintain circulating levels of active molecules to prolong drug effect until the next dose. An important example of a drug that undergoes this is the combined oral contraceptive pill.

General and molecular aspects

It is important that nurses involved in medicines management are aware of the sites of action for many commonly used drugs. Drugs exert their effects at molecular (chemical) targets, of which there are many. Below are some of the commonest.

Receptors

The plasma membrane of a human cell is selectively permeable in that it helps control what moves in and out of the cell. The cell membrane consists of a thin structured bilayer of phospholipids and protein molecules. The surfaces of plasma membranes are generally studded with proteins that perform different functions, like the reception of nutrients. In biochemistry these protein molecules are referred to as *receptors*. Molecules which bind to these receptors are called *ligands*. Examples of ligands are neurotransmitters, hormones or drugs.

A large number of drugs, which are clinically effective, exert their action by interaction with receptors. Examples include:

- ligand-gated ion channels (ionotropic receptors) such as the $GABA_A$ receptor, which binds benzodiazepines;
- G-protein coupled receptors such as adrenoceptors;
- kinase-linked receptors such as the insulin receptor;
- nuclear receptors such as the thyroid receptor.

Ion channels

Ion channels provide receptors which drugs can interact with. Drug actions at ion channels can take two forms (see Figure 1.1). The first form are known as *channel blockers*, whereby the drug blocks permeation of the channel, and the second are *channel modulators* whereby the drug binds to a receptor site within the ion channel and modulates permeation of the channel. This can happen by the drug altering the channel's response to its normal mediator.

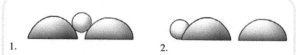

In 1. we see a drug blocking the permeation of the actual ion channel itself.

In 2. we see a drug binding to the channel but not sitting within the channel itself.

Figure 1.1 Drug binding at ion channels

Enzymes

Enzymes are biological catalysts that increase the rate of chemical reactions in the body. They are integral to many normal physiological functions. Many drugs target enzymes to prevent them from carrying out their normal function – for example, Enalopril acts on angiotensin converting enzymes, thereby preventing an increase in blood pressure.

Transport systems

These are also known as carrier molecule interactions. In some transmitter systems, there is normal physiological recycling of the transmitters, such as serotonin. After the release of serotonin from a neurone, it is taken back up by that same neurone using a serotonin-selective re-uptake system. The drug fluoxetine blocks the uptake transporter for serotonin as its mode of action. This results in an increased level of serotonin in the neuronal synapse. This mechanism has an onward effect which facilitates an increase in mood and makes fluoxetine and drugs similar to it good antidepressants.

Drug action

The time to the onset of drug action involves delivery of the drug to its site of action. This is largely controlled by:

- route of administration;
- rate of absorption;
- manner of distribution.

These are important considerations, as often we want the drug to have its effect within a certain time frame. We can speed up the time to the onset of drug action in many ways. If the drug is given orally, we can use liquid or dispersible formulations instead of regular tablets. If drug action is needed more quickly, we can use the intramuscular (IM) or intravenous (IV) route as necessary. For example, if a patient requires pain relief following myocardial infarction they would be given intravenous morphine rather than an oral preparation.

It is also possible to delay drug onset or prolong the effect by using enteric-coated or slow release preparations orally, or by using transdermal or subcutaneous (SC) routes. For example, people suffering with chronic pain from conditions such as rheumatoid arthritis may be given analgesia in the form of a transdermal patch. This is much preferred by the patient as it decreases the amount of oral analgesia required.

The duration of drug effect relates to the time it takes for the drug to be removed from its site of action. This is largely controlled by:

- rate of hepatic metabolism;
- rate of renal excretion.

It is important to be aware of the duration a drug will have its effect for. Drug companies do extensive studies to determine this information. They use the data they obtain to decide upon dosing schedules. It is vital that nurses know the normal dosing schedules for the drugs they are administering (this can easily be found in the British National Formulary – BNF) so that the correct regimen is implemented. Drugs need to be given more than once to have continued effect. Some drugs need to be given daily, while others need to be given two, three or four times per day to maintain effective action.

First pass metabolism

Some drugs undergo destruction by *first pass metabolism*. When absorbed through the stomach after oral administration, the drugs enter blood vessels which go directly to the liver. We call this

the *portal circulation*. This means that drugs which are largely destroyed by liver enzyme systems will not enter the general systemic circulation. An example of such a drug is glyceryl trinitrate (GTN) which is metabolized completely by the liver at this stage. This is why you will find GTN being given via routes other than orally.

The concept of affinity

Drugs have what is termed an *affinity* for their receptors, or chemical targets. This is a measure of how well a drug can bind to its chemical target. The tighter the bond, the better the drug action. Some drugs have a higher affinity for their chemical targets than others. Those with a higher affinity will bind first, in preference to any other drug molecule present. Some drugs have a higher affinity for their targets than even the normal physiological molecule. This can be very useful in drug action, especially where the normal molecule is abundant and causing the problem or symptom the patient is experiencing. Higher affinity means that even small amounts of the drug will bind preferentially.

Agonistic and antagonistic drug action

Drugs can either be *agonists* or *antagonists* at their target sites. This is best explained using receptors as an example (see Figure 1.2). When agonists or antagonists bind to receptors they are said to *occupy* the receptor site. The amount of drug occupying the receptor site relates to the magnitude of response to the drug itself. In simple terms the more of an agonist drug occupying a receptor, the greater the response.

Agonists are drugs that bind to their targets and form a drug-receptor complex. Agonists activate the receptors to produce a response (known as *full agonists*) and have what is termed *positive efficacy*. Antagonists are drugs that bind to their targets and form a drug receptor complex, but without causing activation or response. They can block the receptor to its endogenous activator, thereby blocking normal function. They have what is termed *zero*

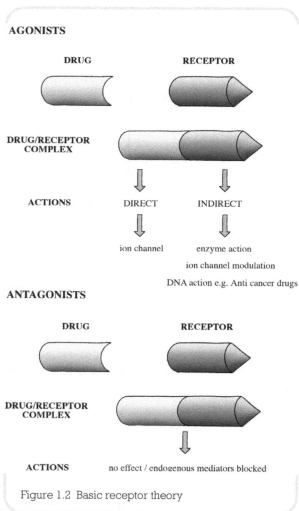

Figure 1.2 Basic receptor theory

efficacy. Receptor occupancy by antagonists is important if the drug is a competitive antagonist – i.e. it competes for occupancy with another drug or with the receptor's normal mediator. The amount of drug occupying will determine any response.

This is a simplistic view of the concepts of agonism and antagonism as the response of a drug at its chemical target is actually graded.

For agonists we have:

- **Partial agonists:** drugs that bind to their targets and activate them to produce a response which is less than that we would expect from a full agonist. They have what is termed *partial efficacy*.

- **Inverse agonists:** drugs that bind to their targets and can reduce the normal activity of that chemical target. They have what is termed *negative efficacy*.

For antagonists we have:

- **Competitive antagonists:** drugs that bind to the chemical targets and prevent activation by the normal target agent.
- **Non-competitive antagonists:** drugs that do not necessarily bind to the chemical target but at a point in the chain of events block target activation.

Drug specificity

Very few drugs are specific for their intended targets within the body. A prescriber will give a drug with a specific action in mind, for example salbutamol. Salbutamol is a beta$_2$ adrenoceptor agonist. This means it has its main action at beta$_2$ adrenoceptors in the bronchi. This gives us its desired effect as a bronchodilator which eases breathing in asthma. However the action of salbutamol is not that specific and can act on other beta$_2$ adrenoceptors in the body as well as on beta adrenoceptors, especially if given in higher doses leading to increased receptor occupancy. This is the reason that some of the side-effects of drugs can be seen. In the case of salbutamol, action at other beta adrenoceptors can lead to palpitations and increased occupancy at non-bronchial beta adrenoceptors can cause tremor.

Basic introduction to units and conversions

Nurses need to be able to make accurate drug calculations in order to safely administer drugs to their patients. It is therefore important that student nurses begin to engage with mathematics early in their education. This brief introduction is aimed at motivating you to engage with other purpose-designed texts to help you develop your skills to the required level.

Box 1.2 Equivalencies of weight

UNIT	SYMBOL	EQUIVALENT	SYMBOL
1 kilogram	kg	1000 grams	g
1 gram	g	1000 milligrams	mg
1 milligram	mg	1000 micrograms	mcg or µg
1 microgram	mcg	1000 nanograms	ng

Before performing many drug calculations you will need to convert the numbers you use in the calculation so that they all appear in the same units. You should be familiar with the units in Box 1.2 as they are the most common in drug calculation.

To convert from a smaller unit (e.g. a gram) to a larger unit (e.g. a kilogram), divide by 1000, so:

$$5000g \div 1000 = 5kg$$

To convert from a larger unit (e.g. a gram) to a smaller unit (e.g. a milligram), multiply by 1000, so:

$$5g \times 1000 = 5000mg$$

It is important to be comfortable with unit conversions before progressing to using a drug calculation formula. Practise some conversions before you move on.

Basic formula
There is more than one way to do a drug calculation, but the simplest and most widely used method is the basic formula shown here:

$$\frac{D \times Q}{H} = X$$

Where:

- D = desired dose
- H = strength available

- Q = quantity or unit of measure (for tablets Q =1, for liquids Q can vary)
- X = dose to be determined/amount to be given

The steps for using the basic formula method are as follows:

- first, memorize the formula;
- remember to convert all the units to same system and size;
- place all of the unit information into the correct position within the basic formula;
- calculate your answer;
- label all answers (e.g. tablets, capsules, ml).

Here are some examples.
The doctor orders a dose of 0.05mg to be given orally
You have 25 microgram tablets
How many tablets should you give?

$$\frac{50}{25} \times 1 = X$$

$$\frac{2}{1} \times 1 = 2$$

$$X = 2 \text{ tablets}$$

The patient requires 400mg of liquid to be given orally
You have 250mg in 5ml of solution

What volume of drug should be given?

$$\frac{400}{250} \times 5 = X$$

$$\frac{8}{5} \times 5 = 8$$

$$X = 8ml$$

The patient needs 240mg of drug D by injection
150mg in 5ml of liquid is available
How many ml will you administer?

The dose has to be given at a rate of 1ml every 30 seconds: how long will each dose last?

$$\frac{240}{150} \times 5 = X$$

$$\frac{24}{15} \times 5 = 8ml \text{ to be given}$$

1 ml every 30 seconds = 2ml every minute

$$\frac{8}{2} = 4 \text{ minutes}$$

You should now be able to attempt the practice questions at the end of this and each relevant chapter.

Case studies

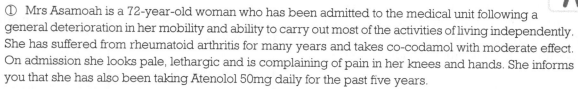

① Mrs Asamoah is a 72-year-old woman who has been admitted to the medical unit following a general deterioration in her mobility and ability to carry out most of the activities of living independently. She has suffered from rheumatoid arthritis for many years and takes co-codamol with moderate effect. On admission she looks pale, lethargic and is complaining of pain in her knees and hands. She informs you that she has also been taking Atenolol 50mg daily for the past five years.

Following a discussion with her daughter, you learn that she has recently commenced a course of trimethoprim to treat a urinary tract infection but has been reluctant to take it as she claims that she has too many tablets to take and they tend to get stuck when swallowing.

● What information from Mrs Asamoah's assessment could you now obtain which would help you identify factors influencing the absorption and distribution of the medication she is taking?

② Mr Mambety is a 42-year-old man who is recovering from emergency gastric surgery. He has a history of heavy drinking and cigarette smoking. His post-operative pain is being controlled by a patient-controlled analgesic device and he is beginning to mobilize with assistance.

● What factors may influence Mr Mambety's ability to metabolize and excrete any drugs he is prescribed during his post-operative recovery?

Key learning points

Introduction

➢ Pharmacology is the study of drugs.
➢ Pharmacodynamics is the effect that drugs have on the body.
➢ Pharmacokinetics is the effect the body has on the drugs.
➢ Pharmacokinetics includes absorption, distribution, metabolism and excretion of drugs.

→

←

Absorption

➤ The main factor which relates to absorption of drugs is the route of administration.
➤ Physiological considerations in absorption are blood flow, total surface area, time of arrival of the drug and time of drug at absorption site.
➤ Other considerations for absorption are solubility, chemical stability and how soluble the drug is in lipids.

Distribution

➤ Drugs are distributed into major body fluids (e.g. plasma).
➤ Specific tissues may take up certain drugs (e.g. iodine is taken up by the thyroid gland).
➤ Drug distribution is affected by the extent that the drug binds to plasma proteins.
➤ Drug distribution is affected by barriers (e.g. the placenta and the BBB).

Biotransformation

➤ This is a process of metabolizing drugs in the body.
➤ It occurs mainly in the liver and is therefore often called hepatic metabolism.
➤ Some drugs are given that are activated by this hepatic metabolism. These are called pro-drugs.
➤ Drug metabolism is split into two phases in the liver.
➤ An example of phase I metabolism would be oxidation.
➤ An example of phase II metabolism would be conjugation.

Excretion

➤ Excretion includes renal elimination and faecal elimination.
➤ The main method of renal elimination is by active glomerular filtration.
➤ Drugs can also be eliminated by passive methods in the distal tubules.
➤ Drugs can be eliminated from the body in bile and so removed in the faeces.

General and molecular aspects

➤ Drugs exert their effects at molecular (chemical) targets (e.g. adrenaline receptors).
➤ Drugs can also act by stopping or partially stopping important ions entering the cell (e.g. calcium channel blockers).
➤ Drugs can interfere with enzymes that are produced by the body.
➤ Drugs can work on the transport of chemicals into and out of cells.

Drug action

➤ Drug action relies on route of administration, rate of absorption and manner of distribution.
➤ The duration of drug effect involves how quickly it is removed from the body.

→

←
- ➢ Some drugs when absorbed from the stomach enter the portal circulation and pass through the liver. This is called the first pass effect.
- ➢ Drug action can also be affected by drug affinity.
- ➢ The greater the affinity the better the drug action.

Agonistic and antagonistic drug action

- ➢ Agonists activate receptors to produce a response.
- ➢ Antagonists bind with receptors but do not activate them or cause a response. They can actually block the activation of receptors.
- ➢ Partial agonists produce a response. However, this is less than would be expected by a full agonistic drug.
- ➢ Inverse agonists are drugs which can reduce the normal activity of the cell.
- ➢ Competitive antagonists are drugs that prevent activation of the cell by their normal agent.
- ➢ Non-competitive antagonists are drugs that may block the receptor but not in a permanent way.

Calculations

1   How many micrograms are in 2mg?

2   How many grams are in 600mg?

3   How many milligrams are in 1.2g?

4   Which strength is the weakest: 1 in 100, 1 in 1000 or 1 in 10,000?

5   If a patient has a fluid intake of 30ml each hour, how much fluid (in ml) have they had after 12 hours?

6   A doctor has prescribed 0.25mg of digoxin. You have 125 microgram tablets in stock. How many should you give?

7   How many 25mg tablets should be administered for a prescribed dose of 0.05g?

For further assistance with calculations, please see Meriel Hutton's *Essential Calculation Skills for Nurses, Midwives and Healthcare Practitioners* (Open University Press 2009).

Multiple choice questions

Try answering these multiple choice questions to test what you have learned from reading this chapter. You can check your answers on page 197.

1 A drug that binds to a cell receptor and affects a response is called

a) An agonist
b) An antagonist
c) A receptor blocker
d) A channel blocker

2 Most drugs and metabolites are excreted by

a) The kidneys
b) The lungs
c) Bile
d) Saliva

3 The four processes in pharmacokinetics are

a) Stomach, liver, kidney and lungs
b) Receptors, ion channels, transport systems and enzymes
c) Administration, absorption, metabolism and elimination
d) Absorption, distribution, metabolism and excretion

4 Pharmacodynamics is defined as

a) The effect our body has on drugs
b) The action of the liver on drug molecules
c) The effect a drug has on our bodies
d) The movement of a drug around the body

5 The main method of renal elimination of a drug is by

a) Passive distal excretion
b) Active glomerular filtration
c) Selective reabsorption
d) Active secretion into the collecting duct

→

←

6 How many phases of hepatic metabolism are there?

a) 1
b) 2
c) 4
d) 10

7 What route should drugs subject to first pass metabolism *not* be given by?

a) IV
b) IM
c) Sublingual
d) Oral

8 Which of the following is a plasma protein?

a) Prostacyclin
b) Albumin
c) Protamine
d) Meatamine

9 A pro-drug is

a) A drug given to promote growth
b) A drug given in its active form
c) A drug given to prevent metabolism of another drug
d) A drug given in its inactive form, requiring metabolism

10 An antagonist can be

a) Competitive and non-competitive
b) Competitive and complimentary
c) Competitive and comparative

Recommended further reading

Beckwith, S. and Franklin, P. (2007) *Oxford Handbook of Nurse Prescribing*. Oxford: Oxford University Press.

Brenner, G.M. and Stevens, C.W. (2006) *Pharmacology*, 2nd edn. Philadelphia, PA: Saunders Elsevier.

Clayton, B.D. (2009) *Basic Pharmacology for Nurses*, 15th edn. St Louis, MO: Mosby Elsevier.

Coben, D. and Atere-Roberts, E. (2005) *Calculations for Nursing and Healthcare*, 2nd edn. Basingstoke: Palgrave Macmillan.

Downie, G., Mackenzie, J. and Williams, A. (2007) *Pharmacology and Medicines Management for Nurses*, 4th edn. Edinburgh: Churchill Livingstone.

Gatford, J.D. and Phillips, N. (2006) *Nursing Calculations*, 7th edn. Edinburgh: Churchill Livingstone Elsevier.

Karch, A.M. (2008) *Focus on Nursing Pharmacology*, 4th edn. Philadelphia, PA: Lippincott Williams & Wilkins.

Lapham, R. and Agar, H. (2003) *Drug Calculations for Nurses: A Step-by-step Approach*, 2nd edn. London: Arnold.

Simonson, T., Aarbakke, J., Kay, I., Coleman, I., Sinnott, P. and Lyssa, R. (2006) *Illustrated Pharmacology for Nurses*. London: Hodder Arnold.

Trounce, J. (2000) *Clinical Pharmacology for Nurses*, 16th edn. New York: Churchill Livingstone.

Adverse drug reactions and interactions

2

Chapter contents

Learning objectives
Introduction
Main mechanisms of drug interactions
  Absorption
  Distribution
  Metabolism
  Excretion
Adverse drug reactions
  Type A: augmented
  Type B: bizarre
Clinical significance of drug interactions to the patient
  Type A ADR
  Type B ADR
  Pharmacovigilance
  The yellow card system

Major groups of drugs involved in adverse drug reactions
Steps in minimizing the effects of adverse drug reactions
  Anaphylaxis
  Treatment
Age-related adverse drug reactions
  Absorption
  Distribution
  Metabolism
  Excretion
Case studies
Key learning points
Multiple choice questions
Recommended further reading

Learning objectives

After studying this chapter you should be able to:

- Convey the importance of recognizing adverse drug reactions and interactions.
- Describe why drug interactions occur in absorption, distribution, metabolism and excretion of drugs.
- Explain what is meant by the terms 'enzyme inducer' and 'inhibitor'.
- Define the term adverse drug reaction.
- Give two examples of different drug reactions.
- Define pharmacovigilance.
- Outline the use of the yellow card system.
- Be aware of anaphylaxis.
- List three common drugs which are frequently implicated in drug reactions.
- Discuss the steps taken in minimizing drug interactions in patient care.
- Describe why elderly people and children are at a higher risk of drug interaction than other age groups.

Introduction

The aim of this chapter is to introduce you to the concepts of adverse drug reactions and drug interactions and side-effects. According to the Department of Health (DH), between 5 and 17 per cent of hospital admissions are associated with adverse drug reactions (DH 2001). The likelihood of drug interactions and adverse reactions is increased in patients on more than one medicine and higher in those who take more than four medications (polypharmacy). The incidence is also increased in elderly patients. As many elderly people are on many medicines, it can be seen that they as a group are often at a higher risk of interactions and adverse reactions.

Main mechanisms of drug interactions

Drug interactions can be described as being:

- pharmacokinetic; and
- pharmacodynamic.

Pharmacokinetic interactions can occur in any of the four pharmacokinetic processes:

- absorption;
- distribution;
- metabolism;
- excretion.

Absorption

The most common absorption interactions occur when medicines are taken by the oral route. Many drugs require precise conditions for optimal absorption in the stomach and upper gastrointestinal (GI) tract. Anything which disrupts these conditions can affect drug absorption. Examples include:

- Taking medication with or after a meal: the presence of food in the stomach can delay drug absorption. Sometimes we use this to our advantage, but some drugs need to be taken on an empty stomach.

- Taking medication at the same time as an antacid preparation. Antacids such as Gaviscon coat the stomach and delay drug absorption, so taking them at the same time as some drugs must be avoided.
- Crushing or splitting tablets. Some tablets need to travel intact through the stomach before being absorbed optimally in the small intestine, or have a coating which delays their absorption. By crushing or splitting tablets we may change the rate of absorption of these drugs.

Clinical tip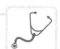

You should not be crushing or tampering with tablets or capsules: many are especially designed to be absorbed in a specific manner in a specific time frame. If in doubt over how the medicine can be given please consult your pharmacist.

The main message is to always follow any special instructions given with oral medicines to ensure optimal absorption.

Distribution

Some drugs are bound to plasma proteins during their distribution through body fluids. The efficiency of a drug can be affected by the degree to which it binds to proteins within the blood plasma. The less a drug binds to a plasma protein, the more efficient it is in diffusing and crossing cell membranes. An example of a common blood protein that drugs can bind to would be albumin. Due to protein binding of a drug, the drug exists in two forms, namely protein bound and unbound (free), the unbound being the active component of the drug. The bound portion remains inactive unless displaced from the protein. Any medications that may displace other medicines from plasma proteins could change the level of free drug in the plasma. Drugs with this sort of interaction are usually listed as incompatible in Appendix 1 of the BNF.

Clinical tip

When working in the clinical setting it is important to be thinking of the age of the person you are dealing with. For example, neonates, infants and older people have a reduced amount of plasma proteins, therefore doses of drugs in these patients should reflect physiological differences.

Metabolism

Some drugs can interfere with the effectiveness of drug metabolizing enzymes in the liver. This can have one of two effects:

1. **Enzyme inducer:** this is where the drug increases the effectiveness of the enzyme and metabolizes more quickly. This means that the effectiveness of other drugs and their duration of action may be reduced.

2. **Enzyme inhibitor:** this is where the drug decreases the effectiveness of the enzyme and metabolizes more slowly. This means that the effectiveness of other drugs and their duration of action may be increased.

Drugs which modify metabolizing enzymes should be given with caution to patients on other medicines, and effects should be monitored. The daily presence of the pharmacist on the ward, monitoring prescriptions, while liaising with both the medical and nursing team, is of great importance in recognizing any such problems.

Clinical tip

When nursing neonates and infants you will notice that certain drugs are given at a reduced level. This is because of the immaturity of the liver to metabolize drugs.

Excretion

Relatively few drugs have a dramatic effect on drug excretion. Non-steroidal anti-inflammatory drugs (NSAIDs) can affect the kidney tubule and modify the excretion and reabsorption of some drugs. Pharmacodynamic interactions are more common and come into two categories.

1. **Additive effects of drugs with similar actions.** For example, giving an angiotensin-converting enzyme (ACE) inhibitor (e.g. Lisinopril) with a diuretic (e.g. Bendroflumethazide) may lead to an adverse drop in blood pressure.

2. **Competing effects of drugs with opposite actions.** For example, giving a beta blocker drug for hypertension (e.g. Propranalol) to an asthmatic patient may render their beta agonist drug (e.g. salbutamol) ineffective in managing their asthma symptoms.

Clinical tip

As a nurse you should keep accurate fluid balance records because patients' renal function needs to be optimal in order to avoid toxicity. Sometimes the first indicator of renal insufficiency is a change in urinary output.

Adverse drug reactions

An adverse drug reaction (ADR) (sometimes called an adverse drug event – ADE) is a reaction that is always unwanted by the patient. It is a negative event following the prescription and administration of a medication. The term ADR differs from a side-effect. This is because some side-effects can be beneficial. The study of ADRs is called *pharmacovigilance*.

The World Health Organization's (WHO) definition of an adverse drug reaction is 'a response to a drug which is noxious and unintended, and which occurs at doses normally used in man for the prophylaxis, diagnosis or therapy of disease or for the modification of a physiological function'. ADRs can be classified according to their cause and there are many categories:

- Type A: augmented effects.
- Type B: bizarre effects.
- Type C: chronic effects.
- Type D: delayed effects.
- Type E: end-of-treatment effects.
- Type F: failure of therapy.

The most common types of ADR are augmented and bizarre.

Type A: augmented

This is where the reaction is an augmentation of the drug's pharmacology. This means we can often predict these reactions from our knowledge of the pharmacodynamic properties of a drug. For example, a patient on an antihypertensive drug may develop dizziness and fainting due to too great a lowering of their blood pressure. Patients on NSAIDs can develop gastric irritation due to the drug's action on protective gastric mucous. These types of reactions are mainly dose dependent: the greater the dose of the drug, the higher the likelihood of adverse reaction. They are the most common ADRs but are associated with lower morbidity and mortality.

Type B: bizarre

This is where the reaction is wholly unexpected and could not be predicted from the pharmacodynamic properties of the drug. An example would be anaphylaxis to any drug, or a red pinprick rash with penicillin. These types of reactions are not dose dependent and can occur even at low starting doses. They are rarer than Type A ADRs but are associated with a higher morbidity and mortality.

Clinical significance of drug interactions to the patient

The significance of a drug reaction to the patient depends on many factors and can determine how health care professionals respond to the reaction. Some patients can tolerate side-effects or ADRs of medications if the benefit of the drug is greater than the inconvenience. When side-effects cannot be tolerated, this may be classed as a Type A ADR.

Type A ADR

If a patient reports an ADR there are a variety of responses. The prescriber should be informed immediately so that appropriate action can be taken. This could include:

- stopping the drug altogether;
- reducing the dose of the drug;
- switching to an alternative drug.

The ADR should always be recorded in the patient's notes. Poor management of ADRs can lead to problems with patients adhering to their medication regimens, so this is an area that should be taken very seriously.

Type B ADR

Type B ADRs are more serious than Type A and require prompt detection and rapid action. The drug suspected of causing this reaction should be withheld and the prescriber informed immediately. Any resuscitative measures should be undertaken at once to prevent serious complications. The drug should be stopped and an alternative found where necessary. This type of ADR should always be recorded in the patient's notes and be easily visible to any future prescriber.

All Type B and many Type A ADRs should be reported to the Medicines & Healthcare Products Regulatory Agency (MHRA) via the yellow card found in the back of the BNF or online. This allows pharmacovigilance and builds up a fuller profile of the drugs.

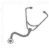

Pharmacovigilance

Pharmacovigilance is the study relating to the detection, assessment, understanding and prevention of adverse drug effects. The origin of the word is a combination of the Greek *pharmakon*, 'drug' and the Latin *vigilare*, 'to keep awake or alert, to keep watch'. In common practice we are mostly concerned with side-effects of medicines that may be intolerable by our patients or cause them to have adverse effects as described above. Pharmacovigilance involves collecting, monitoring, researching, assessing and evaluating information from health care providers and patients on the adverse effects of medications with a view to:

- identifying new information about medicines to inform prescribing practice;
- preventing harm to patients.

A very helpful website in relation to this area can be found at www.mhra.gov.uk/Howweregulate/Medicines/Inspectionandstandards/GoodPharmacovigilancePractice/index.htm.

The yellow card system

The yellow card system is vital in helping the MHRA monitor the safety of the medicines and vaccines on the market. Before a medicine is granted a licence so that it can be made available in the UK, it must pass strict tests and checks to ensure that it is acceptably safe and effective. All effective medicines, however, can cause side-effects (or ADRs, see above), which can range from minor to very serious. Even if it is only a *suspicion* that a medicine or combination of medicines have caused a side-effect, patients and health professionals should send the MHRA a yellow card. Yellow card reports on suspected side-effects are evaluated, together with other sources of information such as clinical trial data, medical literature or data from international medicines regulators, to pinpoint previously unidentified safety issues. The MHRA will take action, whenever necessary, to ensure that medicines are used in a way that minimizes risk, while maximizing patient benefit.

Clinical tip

You must learn to actively listen to the patient and become observant. Look at the prescription chart to see if the person has been prescribed any new medication. Remember to always report any signs or symptoms to the nurse in charge.

Major groups of drugs involved in adverse drug reactions

Some drugs are more likely to cause ADRs than others. This means that their prescribing and administration should be closely monitored. These drug groups include:

- antibiotics;
- antipsychotics;
- NSAIDs;
- drugs with a narrow therapeutic index (e.g. warfarin and Digoxin);
- lithium;
- diuretics;
- benzodiazepines;
- newly-licensed medicines.

Many of these medications have few alternatives that are as effective for some patients, which can mean that reactions may be inevitable.

Steps in minimizing the effects of adverse drug reactions

There are a number of steps that can be taken to minimize or prevent ADRs:

- drugs should only be prescribed for a good indication, particularly during pregnancy;
- a check should be made on all previous medication;
- any previous reactions to medicines should be assessed;

- any non-drug allergies should be identified including food allergies/sensitivities or topical allergies (e.g. sticking plasters);
- other drug use should be verified, including over the counter (OTC) medications, herbal remedies and any illicit or recreational drugs taken;
- age should always be taken into consideration (e.g. is the patient elderly or a young child?);
- check for any hepatic and/or renal disease;
- always maintain yellow card reporting to uphold pharmacovigilance;
- prescribing should be according to any established protocols;
- clear instructions should always be provided regarding medication administration to the patient;
- familiar drugs should be prescribed where possible, as side-effect profiles are better known;
- always inform the patient of possible side-effects to help them identify ADRs.

Nurses have an important role in ADR monitoring. They are well placed to spot ADRs as they are often the people administering the medication to the patient and patients may find it easier to talk to nurses about their medicines during the drug round than to the prescribing doctor. If you suspect a reaction, you must follow local policies and procedures for its reporting and management.

Anaphylaxis

Anaphylaxis is an *acute multi-system severe type I hypersensitivity allergic reaction*. The term comes from the Greek words *ana*, 'against', and *phylaxis*, 'protection'. Anaphylactic shock or true anaphylaxisis is associated with systemic vasodilation that results in low blood pressure. It is also associated with severe bronchoconstriction to the point where the individual finds in increasingly difficult to breathe. Anaphylaxis can present with many different symptoms. These usually develop quickly over a few minutes. The most common systems affected include the skin, the respiratory system, the gas-

trointestinal system, the heart and vasculature, and the central nervous system. Anaphylaxis can occur in response to any allergen. Common triggers include insect bites or stings, foods, medications and latex. The most common medicines to trigger anaphylaxis are antibiotics, aspirin, ibuprofen and other analgesics.

Treatment

The Resuscitation Council (UK) issues guidelines for the treatment and management of anaphylaxis (Resuscitation Council 2008). The key points are:

Treatment of an anaphylactic reaction should be based on general life support principles:

- use the airway, breathing, circulation, disability, exposure (ABCDE) approach to recognize and treat problems;
- call for help early;
- treat the greatest threat to life first;
- initial treatments should not be delayed by the lack of a complete history or definite diagnosis.

Patients having an anaphylactic reaction in any setting should expect the following as a minimum:

- recognition that they are seriously unwell;
- an early call for help;
- initial assessment and treatments based on an ABCDE approach;
- adrenaline therapy if indicated;
- investigation and follow-up by an allergy specialist.

The full guidance can be downloaded from the Resuscitation Council website at www.resus.org.uk/pages/reaction.pdf.

Age-related adverse drug reactions

As previously noted, the elderly and the very young are at a higher risk of drug reactions and should be closely monitored when prescribed medications which have a higher incidence of drug reactions

Box 2.1 Pharmacokinetic features in children and adolescents

Absorption (children and adolescents)	**Distribution (children under 6)**
➢ Delayed gastric emptying ➢ Slower GI transit (longer contact) ➢ Thinner skin ➢ Use of rectal administration	➢ Plasma protein levels lower immediately after birth, especially in premature babies ➢ Presence of bilirubin can affect binding to plasma proteins ➢ More body water for drug distribution
Metabolism (children under 3 months)	**Excretion (children under 6 months)**
➢ Liver maturity happens quickly after birth in term babies, usually by four weeks ➢ Conjugation of bilirubin occurs ➢ Increased clearance after four weeks due to relative liver mass and hepatic blood flow being higher	➢ Glomerular filtration is 40 per cent of adult level at birth ➢ Tubular secretion processes poorly developed ➢ Renal maturity slower than liver, reaching full maturity only after six months in the term infant

or side-effects. The elderly often have changes in sensitivity to drugs due to:

● reductions in drug binding sites;
● impaired organ function (liver/kidneys);
● altered metabolizing enzyme systems in the liver.

All of these can lead to potentiation of drug action which in turn can cause more side-effects.

Medicine-related problems are more likely to be associated with older people who:

● take four or more medicines (polypharmacy);
● take Digoxin, warfarin, NSAIDs, diuretics or benzodiazepines;
● have recently been discharged from hospital;
● have a low level of social support;
● have poor hearing, vision or dexterity;
● experience confusion, disorientation or depression.

Children cannot just be viewed as small adults when it comes to medication. They respond differently to drugs for many reasons, most of which can be related to pharmacokinetics (see Chapter 1; see also Box 2.1).

Absorption

This can be a major factor in drug problems with children under the age of 12. Delayed gastric emptying means drugs taken orally stay in the stomach longer, which can in turn delay the absorption of drugs from the small intestine. Children have a longer GI transit of gut contained materials which means drugs stay in contact with their absorbing sites for longer. Also, young children have trouble swallowing tablets and often cannot tolerate liquid medicines well.

Clinical tip

Drugs are sometimes administered rectally in small children. If drugs are given transdermally, the fact children have thinner skin means that they absorb the drug more quickly by this route.

Distribution

Plasma protein levels are lower immediately after birth, especially in premature babies. This can be a problem in drugs which are extensively bound to plasma proteins. If proteins are reduced there are less sites to bind, which increases the available drug, hence effectively increasing the dose which can lead to Type A reactions.

Metabolism

Children metabolize drugs differently to adults, especially in the first few weeks of life. This can lead to higher levels of an active drug being present for longer and produces a risk of Type A reactions.

Excretion

Children's kidneys are immature at birth and cannot efficiently process drug molecules. This leads to delays in excreting drug molecules which can continue to circulate for longer, again with a risk of Type A reactions.

All of these effects mean that children need lower doses of medicine than adults, not simply because they are smaller, but due to immaturity of many organ systems.

Doses of drugs can be increased at 6 months and slowly raised to adult doses for many drugs by the age of 12, when organ maturity is achieved.

Case studies

① Marek Brodzki is a 19-year-old man who has been newly commenced on antibiotics for a post-operative wound infection. You are helping him to dress when you notice a red pinprick rash all over his upper body. You suspect this has been caused by the antibiotics. What are your responsibilities in this matter and what course of action should be taken regarding:

- the antibiotics;
- recording of the incident;
- prevention of recurrence?

② Sue Kent is an elderly woman on many different medicines to manage her complex health needs. One of her medicines is ibuprofen for her knee pain. She is also on warfarin for her atrial fibrillation. Using the BNF, identify any possible interactions between these drugs and whether or not suitable alternatives or further prescribing may be necessary.

Key learning points

Introduction

➤ Between 5 and 17 per cent of hospital admissions are thought to be associated with adverse drug reactions.
➤ The risk of adverse drug reactions increases with the amount of drugs being taken.
➤ The elderly are a higher risk group.

Main mechanisms of drug interactions

➤ The presence of food in the stomach can delay absorption.

- ➤ Taking medication at the same time as an antacid preparation can affect drug absorption.
- ➤ Crushing or splitting of tablets can affect how they are absorbed by the body.
- ➤ Some drugs can bind to plasma proteins, therefore affecting their distribution in the body.
- ➤ Some drugs increase the effectiveness of enzymes in the liver to break down other drugs more quickly. These are called enzyme inducers.
- ➤ Some drugs cause the enzyme in the liver to decrease, therefore affecting the duration of action of certain drugs. These are called enzyme inhibitors.
- ➤ Very few drugs have dramatic affects on drug excretion.
- ➤ Non-steroidal anti-inflammatory drugs may affect excretion and reabsorption of certain drugs.

Adverse drug reactions

- ➤ An ADR is always a negative event following prescription and administration of a medication.
- ➤ The most common types of ADR are augmented and bizarre.
- ➤ An augmented ADR is often a predictable reaction. These types of reaction are mainly dose dependent.
- ➤ A bizarre ADR is wholly unexpected and could not be predicted from the properties of the drug (e.g. anaphylaxis). These reactions are not dose dependent and are more rare than augmented ADRs.

Clinical significance of drug interactions to the patient

- ➤ When side-effects cannot be tolerated we have a Type A ADR.
- ➤ When a Type A ADR is reported the drug may be stopped, the dose reduced or an alternative drug prescribed.
- ➤ All ADRs should be reported in the patient's documentation.
- ➤ Poor management of ADRs can lead to poor adherence to medication regimes.
- ➤ Type B ADRs require prompt detection and rapid action. The drug should be immediately stopped and an alternative found.
- ➤ All Type B and many Type A ADRs should be reported via the yellow card found in the BNF.
- ➤ Some drugs are more likely to cause ADRs than others (e.g. warfarin).
- ➤ Steps in minimizing the effects of drug interactions should be taken (e.g. check all previous medication).

Age-related adverse drug reactions

- ➤ The elderly and children are at a greater risk of drug reactions.
- ➤ The elderly are often more sensitive to drugs, take more than four medicines and have less social support.
- ➤ Children respond differently to drugs for many reasons, most of which can be related to differences in absorption, distribution, metabolism and excretion of drugs compared with adults.

Multiple choice questions

Try answering these multiple choice questions to test what you have learned from reading this chapter. You can check your answers on page 197.

1 What does ADR stand for?

a) A drug response
b) Adverse drug reaction
c) A dangerous reaction
d) Avoidable drug response

2 What are the two main types of ADR?

a) Accidental and bizarre
b) Accelerated and bad
c) Augmented and bizarre
d) Absolute and beneficial

3 Drug interactions can be

a) Predictable and non-predictable
b) Pharmacokinetic and pharmacodynamic
c) Found in polypharmacy
d) All of the above are true

4 The elderly are

a) Not affected by ADRs
b) All on four or more medicines
c) Unable to tolerate side-effects
d) More susceptible to drug interactions

5 Children react to drug therapy differently to adults because

a) They have immature liver and kidneys
b) They are smaller
c) They may not be able to tolerate more than one drug
d) All of the above are true

6 Side-effects of drugs

a) Can always be predicted
b) Can always be avoided
c) Can sometimes become ADRs
d) Only happen at high doses

←

7 Pharmacodynamic interactions can occur when

a) Two drugs are given at the same time of day
b) Two drugs are given for the same condition
c) The action of one drug competes with the action of another
d) One drug blocks the absorption of another

8 Which of the following is an *adverse* reaction?

a) Sedation with a sleeping tablet
b) Reduced blood pressure with an antihypertensive drug
c) Nausea with an emetic drug
d) Rash with an antibiotic drug

9 A drug given to prevent an adverse effect is called

a) A pro-drug
b) A prophylactic drug
c) A drug given to prevent metabolism of another drug
d) A placebo

10 Anaphylaxis is an example of

a) A Type B ADR
b) A predictable drug side-effect
c) Polypharmacy
d) A Type A ADR

Recommended further reading

Beckwith, S. and Franklin, P. (2007) *Oxford Handbook of Nurse Prescribing*. Oxford: Oxford University Press.

Brenner, G.M. and Stevens, C.W. (2006) *Pharmacology*, 2nd edn. Philadelphia, PA: Saunders Elsevier.

Clayton, B.D. (2009) *Basic Pharmacology for Nurses*, 15th edn. St Louis, MO: Mosby Elsevier.

Coben, D. and Atere-Roberts, E. (2005) *Calculations for Nursing and Healthcare*, 2nd edn. Basingstoke: Palgrave Macmillan.

DH (Department of Health) (2001) *National Service Framework: Medicines and Older People*. London: DH.

Downie, G., Mackenzie, J. and Williams, A. (2007) *Pharmacology and Medicines Management for Nurses*, 4th edn. Edinburgh: Churchill Livingstone.

Gatford, J.D. and Phillips, N. (2006) *Nursing Calculations*, 7th edn. Edinburgh: Churchill Livingstone Elsevier.

Karch, A.M. (2008) *Focus on Nursing Pharmacology*, 4th edn. Philadelphia, PA: Lippincott Williams & Wilkins.

Lapham, R. and Agar, H. (2003) *Drug Calculations for Nurses: A Step-by-step Approach*, 2nd edn. London: Arnold.

Resuscitation Council UK (2008) *Emergency Treatment of Anaphylactic Reactions: Guidelines for Healthcare Providers*. London: Resuscitation Council UK.

Simonson, T., Aarbakke, J., Kay, I., Coleman, I., Sinnott, P. and Lyssa, R. (2006) *Illustrated Pharmacology for Nurses*. London: Hodder Arnold.

Trounce, J. (2000) *Clinical Pharmacology for Nurses*, 16th edn. New York: Churchill Livingstone.

Local anaesthetics and analgesics

3

Chapter contents

Learning objectives
Introduction
Neurones
The nerve impulse
Pain reception
The body's analgesic system
Types of pain
Nociceptive (tissue) pain
Neuropathic (nerve) pain
Local anaesthetics
Mode of action
Preparations of local anaesthetics
Topical anaesthesia
Infiltration anaesthesia
Nerve blockade (conduction anaesthesia)
Extradural, epidural and caudal anaesthesia
Spinal anaesthesia
Intravenous local anaesthesia

Unwanted effects of local anaesthetics
The analgesic ladder
Non-steroidal anti-inflammatory drugs
Aspirin
Ibuprofen
Diclofenac
Paracetamol
Opioid analgesics
Morphine
Fentanyl
Codeine
Opioid antagonists
Adjuvant drugs
Case studies
Key learning points
Calculations
Multiple choice questions
Recommended further reading

Learning objectives

After studying this chapter you should be able to:

- Understand how a nerve impulse is initiated and transmitted.
- Describe pain reception, transmission and interpretation.
- Outline the body's analgesic system.
- Discuss the mode of action of local anaesthetic agents.
- Identify the major ways local anaesthetic agents are administered.
- List unwanted effects of local anaesthetic agents.
- Name at least two major drugs from the non-steroidal anti-inflammatory and opiate classifications of analgesics.

- Compare and contrast the mode of action of non-steroidal anti-inflammatory and opioid analgesics.
- Demonstrate knowledge of the unwanted effects of non-steroidal anti-inflammatory and opioid classifications of analgesics.
- State the major opioid antagonist used in clinical practice.
- Define the term 'adjuvant drug'.
- Correctly solve a number of drug calculations with regard to local anaesthetics and analgesic drugs.

Introduction

Pain is a sensation that lets us know about damage occurring to our tissue. It is one of our defence mechanisms and is important to our survival. Therefore, when we consider modifying the experience of pain, it is important to remember that, although distressing and unpleasant, pain has a role to play in protecting us. Having said all this, it is possible to suffer severe pain without any obvious tissue damage or injury – for example, trigeminal neuralgia (severe burning or stabbing pain in the face arising from one of the nerves carrying sensation). On the other hand, pain may become a dominant feature in a person's life long after tissues have healed – for example, phantom limb pains. It is also possible that tissue damage in one part of the body can lead to pain being perceived in another part of the body. This is called *referred pain*.

Pain is therefore a very difficult concept to define. As it becomes more chronic in nature (i.e. more than six months in duration) it begins to affect all activities of daily living, not just from a physical but also from a psychological and sociological perspective. The nurse has a unique role to play in minimizing pain for patients. In order to carry out this role effectively, nurses need to have some understanding of the drugs used in pain relief.

However, before we plunge headlong into the classification of local anaesthetics and analgesics, we need to remind ourselves of the basic principles of, first, the initiation and conduction of nerve impulses, and second, the body's pain pathways and analgesic system.

Neurones

Neurones are specialized cells whose function is to transmit messages. A neurone has branch-like processes called dendrites that convey incoming messages (action potentials) towards the cell body (see Figure 3.1). The cell body houses the nucleus and therefore is the metabolic centre. Conducting impulses away from the cell body we have structures known as *axons*, which terminate in *axon terminals*. Housed in the axon terminals are hundreds of small sacs (vesicles), which contain *neurotransmitters*. The nerve impulse therefore travels from the dendrites along the axon and finishes at the axon terminal where the impulse stimulates the release of the neurotransmitter.

Quite a number of neurones are covered with a substance called myelin, formed by supporting cells called Schwann cells, which wrap themselves around the axon. The myelin covering acts as an insulator for the nerve and also affects the speed at which messages can travel along individual neurones.

Neurones carrying messages from the internal organs and skin into the central nervous system are called *sensory (afferent) neurones*. Conversely, neurones carrying messages out of the central nervous system to the muscles, glands and internal organs are called *motor (efferent) neurones*.

The nerve impulse

At rest, the inside of a neurone has a negative charge compared to the outside, which is positive. This is because the inside of a neurone carries a lot of negatively charged particles called *anions*. Anions are large particles that find difficulty in moving

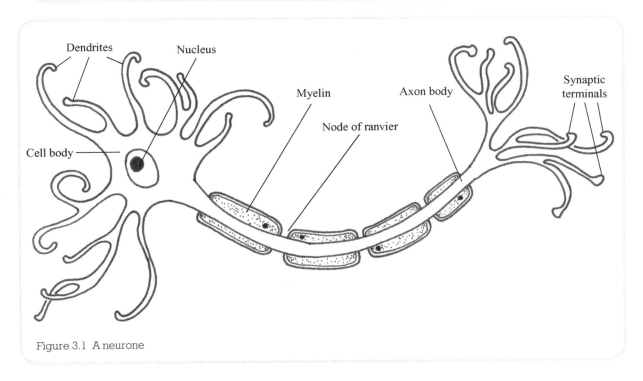

Figure 3.1 A neurone

through the wall of the neurone. The outside of the neurone on the other hand contains lots of positively charged particles called *cations*. The major cation in our discussion here is sodium.

In order to trigger the sensation of pain, the inside of the neurone must become positively charged as compared to the outside. Chemicals liberated by damaged tissue (e.g. bradykinin, histamine, serotonin, potassium and other proteolytic enzymes) bring about a change in the neuronal membrane, allowing sodium to pass into the neurone. As the sodium enters, the membrane becomes even more permeable to sodium. This continues until the inside of the neurone is positively charged in relation to the outside. This build up of positively charged sodium is termed *depolarization*.

At the synapse, where one neurone meets another, neurotransmitters must be released in order to stimulate the next neurone to continue to pass the message onwards. This process is important when considering analgesics and how they work. Once the neurone has converted to a positive environment, calcium channels in the membrane open, so allowing calcium to enter. The influx of cal-

cium attracts small sacs called synaptic vesicles, which are full of neurotransmitters, towards the synapse. When these vesicles reach the synapse they fuse with the neurone membrane and pour their cargo of neurotransmitter into the synapse itself (see Figure 3.2).

The neurotransmitters which are important in the pain pathway are substance P, neurokinin A and B, and glutamate. Once the neurotransmitter attaches itself to receptors on the other side of the synapse, this neurone then becomes permeable to sodium and the process continues (see Figure 3.3).

Having discussed the initiation and transmission of a nerve impulse, we need now to consider the body's pain pathways.

Pain reception

Pain is received via specialist receptors called *nociceptors*, which are free nerve endings that lie in the tissues. They are most plentiful in the skin; as you move deeper into the tissues of the body, they become fewer in number. Nociceptors are stimulated by mechanical, thermal and chemical means and

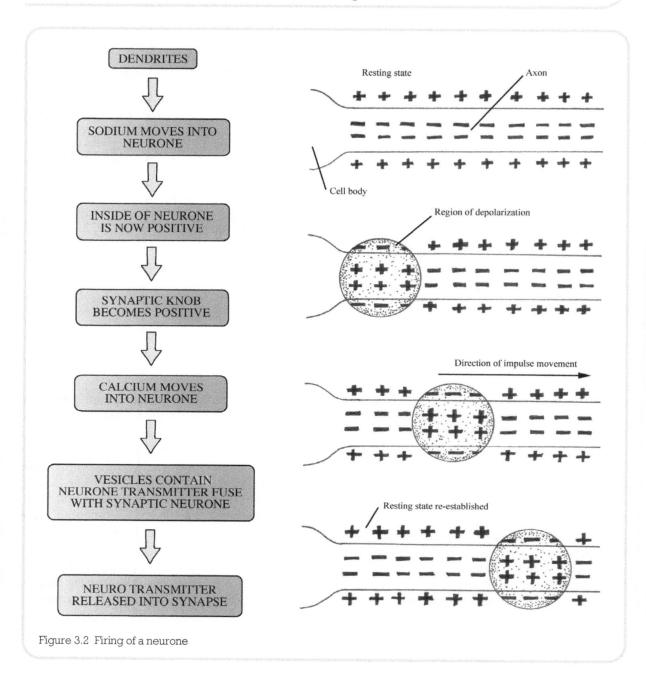

Figure 3.2 Firing of a neurone

have a high threshold. This means that only stimuli indicating some degree of tissue damage are perceived as pain. For example, if you were to apply a heat pad to your skin you would not stimulate your nociceptors until it reached a heat of 40°C, at which point you would feel a sensation of pain. Nociceptors are *non-adapting*, which means they are stimulated at the same level of intensity each time the threshold level is reached. In other words, you do not raise the threshold at which the nociceptors are stimulated just because the pain is constant. This is an important aspect to our survival.

In addition to noxious stimuli like heat and pressure, nociceptors can become sensitive to a variety

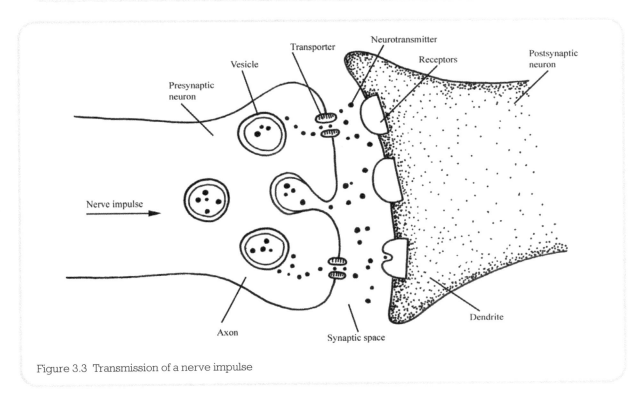

Figure 3.3 Transmission of a nerve impulse

of chemicals which are present after local tissue injury. These substances include potassium, serotonin, bradykinin, histamine and prostaglandins. Prostaglandins are normally produced by the body to ensure the smooth running of our internal environment (homeostasis). They are of particular importance when considering certain medicines, such as NSAIDs.

Painful stimuli are received by the nociceptors and then transmitted by two different types of nerve fibres: A delta fibres and C fibres. A delta fibres are myelinated fibres, small in diameter, which are stimulated by mechanical means. A myelinated nerve is one covered by a fatty insulating substance called myelin. As the fibres are myelinated they convey impulses very quickly. Stimulation of these fibres leads to sharp prickling pain that the person can easily localize. C fibres are also small diameter fibres but are unmyelinated and so convey impulses more slowly, resulting in a 'burning' or 'aching' pain which is harder to pinpoint. It will tend to be more general in nature, and a good example is abdominal pain.

Both A delta and C fibres synapse with the next neurone in the pathway in the dorsal horn of the spinal cord. It is in this area of the dorsal horn (i.e. the substantia gelatinosa) that Melzack and Wall (1965) proposed a gate-controlled entry for the sensation of pain into the central nervous system. If the gate was opened a person would perceive pain; if the gate was closed a person would not.

The sensation of pain is then carried by what are referred to as the *spinothalamic tracks*, which carry impulses from the spinal cord up to the thalamus. One track carries information from the A delta fibres and the other from the C fibres. These tracks once again synapse in the thalamus and the impulses are conveyed to a number of areas including the sensory cortex, where they are interpreted as pain (see Figures 3.4 and 3.5).

The body's analgesic system

As with other sensory systems in the body, the pain pathway has a descending mechanism (see

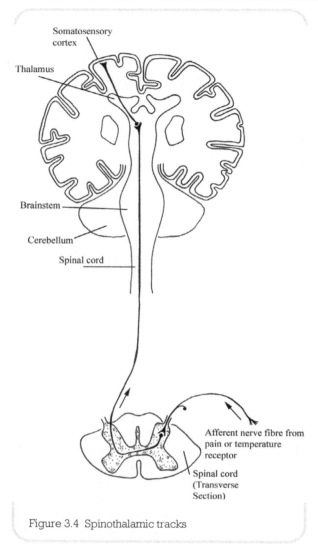

Figure 3.4 Spinothalamic tracks

The PAG connects to an area in the medulla called the nucleus raphe magnus (NRM). This in turn sends fibres down the spinal cord and they interact at the dorsal horn. Therefore, higher brain centres have the infrastructure to open or close the gate to pain in the substantia gelatinosa.

While we suggested that substance P was a neurotransmitter which has been implicated in the transmission of pain, there are also a number of peptides that have been discovered which have been implicated in the brain's analgesic system. The three families of these peptides are *endorphins*, *dynorphins* and *enkephalins*. The discovery of these proteins has been very valuable in our understanding of why opiate drugs, such as morphine, have such a unique effect on the body.

Types of pain

Nociceptive (tissue) pain

Nociceptive pain results from tissue damage. Intact pain pathways report this damage via their neurons, and pain is experienced. Nociceptive pain can further be subdivided into *somatic* and *visceral* (gut) pain. It can be experienced as sharp, dull, or aching. There may be radiation of the pain, especially visceral pain, but it will not be in a direct nerve distribution. For example, gall bladder pain can radiate to the tip of the left scapula. Nociceptive pain generally responds to NSAIDs and opioids, both of which will be introduced further in this chapter. Conditions associated with inflammation, bone pain, and joint disease are particularly responsive to NSAIDs.

Neuropathic (nerve) pain

Neuropathic pain may occur when there is either damage to or dysfunction of nerves in the peripheral or central nervous system. This results in faulty signals being sent to the brain and experienced as pain. Neuropathic pain can be either peripheral (outside the central nervous system) or central (spinal cord and brain) in origin. Examples of neuropathic pain include diabetic neuropathy, trigeminal neuralgia, postherpetic zoster pain (peripheral pains) and thalamic pain syndrome (a central pain).

Figure 3.6). This mechanism constitutes the body's attempt to modify the pain we interpret. In other words, it is our inbuilt analgesic system.

This analgesic system commences at an area of the brain called the periaqueductal grey (PAG). This is a tiny part of grey matter that lies in the mid-brain. It receives input from a number of brain areas, among them the hypothalamus, cortex and thalamus. The PAG is thought to be the mechanism by which the gate to pain can be closed. It would certainly explain in physiological terms why psychological approaches to pain management are successful.

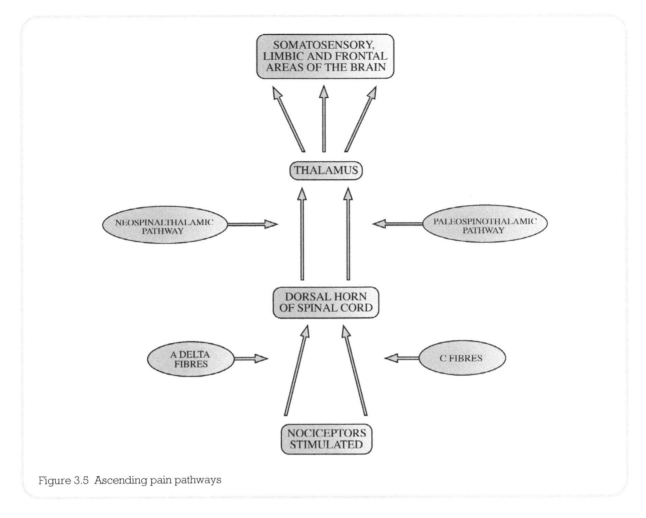

Figure 3.5 Ascending pain pathways

Neuropathic pain frequently exists alongside nociceptive pain. Examples include trauma that damages tissue and nerves, burns (that burn skin as well as nerve endings) and external nerve compression. Examples of the latter include tumours that press on (compress) nerves and the pain of sciatica, caused by herniated intervertebral discs pressing on nerves.

Patients often describe neuropathic pain as a 'burning sensation'. They may also describe it as feeling like an electric shock or lightning bolt. Sometimes stimuli that usually do not cause pain, such as light touch, may elicit a painful response. A light stroke of the cheek that results in the sudden pain of trigeminal neuralgia is an example of this type of pain. Sometimes patients do not describe the sensation as being 'painful' but rather as feeling unpleasantly strange or 'tingly', rather like an arm feels when it wakes up from 'going to sleep'. This is called a dysesthesia. Diabetic neuropathy commonly results in this type of sensation.

Neuropathic pain in the peripheral nervous system frequently follows a nerve distribution. This distribution may follow a particular nerve, as in sciatic pain or trigeminal neuralgia, or may represent the distribution of terminal nerve endings, as in the 'stocking-glove' distribution of peripheral neuropathies. Neuropathic pain is relatively resistant to NSAIDs and opioids, although they may be helpful in certain cases. The other major classes of medications useful for neuropathic pain, tricyclic antidepressants, anticonvulsants

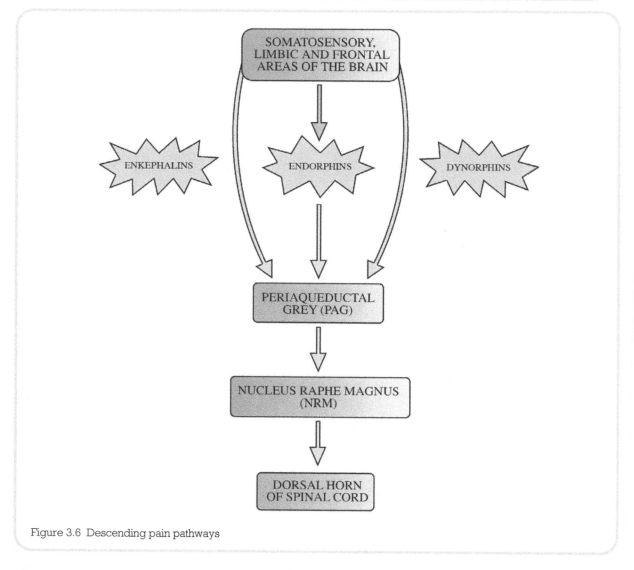

Figure 3.6 Descending pain pathways

and sodium channel blockers are referred to as *adjuvant therapy* which will be discussed later.

Local anaesthetics

Local anaesthetics are analgesic drugs designed to be used clinically to produce a reversible loss of sensation in a particular part of the body. Generally, there are two classes of local anaesthetic: *ester agents*, such as cocaine, procaine and amethocaine, and *amides* such as lignocaine, pilocaine and bupivacaine. The difference between the two comes down to biochemistry.

■ Esters are more unstable in solution than amides and are relatively quickly broken down by enzymes in the plasma. One of the products produced when this group of drugs is broken down is a compound known as para-amino benzoate acid (PABA). Unfortunately, this has been associated with allergic responses and hypersensitivity reactions.

- The amide group do not have any of the above problems. Therefore, you may find in practice that you come across more drugs from this class.

Mode of action

Local anaesthetics block the sodium channels in the neuronal membrane. We can quite clearly link this back to our discussions on initiating an action potential. If sodium cannot move over the semi-permeable membrane then the inside of the neurone does not become depolarized – i.e. the environment remains negative rather than becoming positively charged. Local anaesthetics tend to block conduction more effectively in small diameter nerve fibres and this makes them perfect for the A delta and C fibres described earlier. Therefore, pain is blocked more effectively than other sensations, such as touch. Also, this makes it possible for the doctor to provide a good level of analgesia without too much loss of motor function. You can observe this for yourself in your patients or may even have experienced it following an epidural anaesthetic during labour.

Preparations of local anaesthetics

Local anaesthetics are usually dissolved in a solution which also contains a preservative and fungicide. The dilute preparations are usually presented as percentage solutions of the drug. For example, lignocaine 1 per cent contains 1g of lignocaine in every 100ml. The number of milligrams/millilitres can easily be calculated by multiplying the percentage of the strength by 10. Therefore, a 1 per cent solution of lignocaine contains 10mg of lignocaine to every millilitre of solution.

One of the problems encountered when giving a local anaesthetic is that many of them cause the surrounding vessels to dilate. This leads to rapid absorption of the drug, reducing its effect. For this reason, a vasoconstrictor is sometimes added to increase potency and prolong action. Vasoconstrictors also decrease the chance of systemic side-effects, making local anaesthetics safer. The most common drug added to local anaesthetics is adrenaline.

The effect of vasoconstrictors on the potency and duration of action of local anaesthetics varies according to the drug being given and the site at which it is being used.

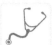

Clinical tip

Solutions containing adrenaline should never be used for infiltration around the penis or in toe blocks, as the constrictive effects could lead to severe ischaemia and necrosis.

Topical anaesthesia

Local anaesthetics are produced that are effective for the skin, eyes, ears, nose and mouth (e.g. pilocaine, lignocaine and amethocaine). When used topically, the onset of action is around 5 to 10 minutes, the drug action lasting between 30 and 60 minutes. This method of application numbs a small area of skin so is ideal for relieving pain from sunburn, minor burns and insect bites. Topical application can also be administered to the surface of the eye allowing certain operative procedures to take place. It must be remembered that these drugs can be absorbed in a significant amount, especially if applied to very vascular areas.

Clinical tip

If you work in paediatric practice, you will come across EMLA cream. This is a cream eutectic mixture of local anaesthetics, which is usually used to provide surface anaesthesia of the skin in children prior to insertion of a cannula. EMLA cream is a mixture of equal proportions of lignocaine and pilocaine. The medicine should be applied to the skin under an occlusive dressing and should be left for 60 minutes before the procedure. Amethocaine gel is an alternative preparation, which may cause some vasodilation, so being advantageous when inserting a needle into a vessel.

Infiltration anaesthesia

This technique is used to provide anaesthesia for minor surgical procedures such as dental work. Lignocaine and pilocaine are again frequently used and the result is that the patient will feel pressure but no pain. The onset of action is very rapid, while the duration depends on the drug being used, pilocaine having the shortest period of action (15 to 30 minutes), while lignocaine provides a moderate length of anaesthesia (60 minutes). Bupivacaine has the longest duration of action, at around 200 minutes. Often the effects of the local anaesthetic continue after the procedure is concluded, so providing extra pain relief. As discussed earlier, the addition of adrenaline will increase the quality and duration of these anaesthetics.

Nerve blockade (conduction anaesthesia)

As the name implies, in conduction anaesthesia, the nerves relating to the area being operated upon are blocked with a local anaesthetic. The blockade may be minor (e.g. intercostals) or deep (e.g. brachial plexus). Drugs such as lignocaine are used for minor blocks and have an onset of 5–10 minutes and duration of 1–2 hours. In a major blockade, the onset can be more variable so communication with the patient is paramount. The local anaesthetic in this case takes a little longer to act (10–15 minutes), but has a more pronounced period of analgesia, at about 3–4 hours. Bupivacaine can be effective for up to 10 hours. The advantages of this approach are that a relatively small amount of the drug can be administered to achieve a wide area of anaesthesia. Nerve blockade can also be used in conjunction with a general anaesthetic to reduce the amount of drugs used in the procedure and the resulting side-effects.

Extradural, epidural and caudal anaesthesia

For these procedures, the local anaesthetic is injected between the dura (the outside covering of the brain and spinal cord) and the periosteum of the bones lining the vertebral cord. Either lignocaine or bupivicaine are used in this technique. The advantage of an epidural approach is that a care-

fully placed needle can achieve a pain-free band from about the mid-chest to the mid-thighs but at the same time allowing the legs to maintain their normal strength. A further local anaesthetic can be administered into a reservoir connected to a fine tube placed in the patient's lower back.

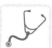

Clinical tip

You may find that the anaesthetist wants to keep the anaesthesia topped up. However, it has been noted that with repeated administration a diminished response may be seen.

Clinical tip

Do not forget that the patient will have loss of other sensations post-procedure so you should monitor their lower limbs for any potential trauma.

Spinal anaesthesia

This is a specialized procedure which anaesthetizes the lower half of the body and does not maintain leg strength: the patient is unable to move their legs. The local anaesthetic in this case is put directly into the cerebrospinal fluid. The drugs are rapidly taken up, which leads to a faster onset and requires a smaller dose. Care must be taken if using this route of administration in pregnant women, as the volume of the subarachnoid space (see Figure 3.7) is diminished; therefore, reduced doses are required.

Intravenous local anaesthesia

This is sometimes referred to as a *Biers block*. First, the limb is elevated to encourage drainage of blood. Further exsanguination is possible by applying a large rubber bandage called an esmachs bandage. A blood pressure cuff would have been

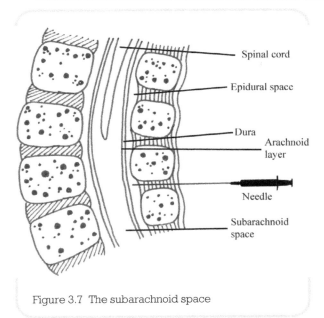

- Spinal cord
- Epidural space
- Dura
- Arachnoid layer
- Needle
- Subarachnoid space

Figure 3.7 The subarachnoid space

applied prior to the procedure and this is now inflated to above the arterial pressure.

The local anaesthetic (pilocaine 40ml of 5 per cent strength) is then injected into a previously cannulated vessel. The anaesthetic agent infiltrates the tissues below the level of the blood pressure cuff. The onset of action is almost immediate, giving excellent anaesthesia for any procedure.

Clinical tip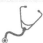

Systemic blood levels of pilocaine are not significant, providing the cuff is not deflated for a period of 15 minutes following initial injection.

Unwanted effects of local anaesthetics

Local anaesthetics are relatively safe as long as they are administered in an appropriate dosage and given into the correct anatomical area. The main areas of unwanted effects from this group of drugs are the central nervous system and the cardiovascular system.

It is not surprising that such drugs have a profound effect on the central nervous system considering their mode of action on cell membranes. Initial mild symptoms may include a feeling of dizziness, leading to sensory disturbances. Severe central nervous system responses to local anaesthetics include major convulsions, followed by acute central nervous system depression indicated by respiratory arrest and coma.

The cardiovascular effects tend to be associated with myocardial depression and vasodilation. The myocardium loses its ability to contract effectively and coupled with the dilation of vessels this leads to a rapid and life-threatening fall in blood pressure.

Clinical tip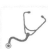

Personnel must always be alert to the possibility of accidental injection into veins and arteries.

A true allergic reaction to a local anaesthetic agent is rare. Some people are sensitive to what are called *parabens* (preservatives in local anaesthetics), albeit rarely. The preservatives, methylparaben or propylparaben, may act as the allergen. The symptoms that occur following a possible allergic reaction to a local anaesthetic agent must be distinguished from toxic reactions due to overdosage (unintended intravenous injection) and reactions occurring as a side-effect of adrenaline (used as an additive).

In the rare event that a patient has sensitivity to a local anaesthetic, skin tests should be undertaken using preparations without parabens. In addition, adrenaline-containing preparations are avoided, as they mask a positive skin test.

The analgesic ladder

Before discussing further analgesics it is useful to consider whether a framework exists to help in planning the pharmacological pathway a patient in pain may tread. The WHO (1966) offers what is commonly known as the *analgesic ladder*. This is a step by step escalation of a variety of analgesics

Box 3.1 Local anaesthetic administration

TOPICAL	Applied directly to the skin, eyes, ears, nose or mouth
INFILTRATION ANAESTHESIA	Applied by penetration of surrounding tissue area
NERVE BLOCKADE	Applied directly to neurone supplying pain sensation to an area of the body
EPIDURAL	Applied to space between the dura and skull
SPINAL	Applied directly into the subarachnoid space
INTRAVENOUS	Applied directly into the vein of a limb

depending upon the severity of pain experienced and is administered in standard doses at regular intervals. Step 1 commences with the use of paracetamol and NSAIDs such as ibuprofen. If the pain continues the patient moves on to Step 2. This step involves giving the patient a weak opioid such as codeine. If the pain is still not controlled, the final step in the ladder is to administer a strong opioid such as morphine. Progress up the ladder frequently involves using analgesic drugs in combination (See Figure 3.8).

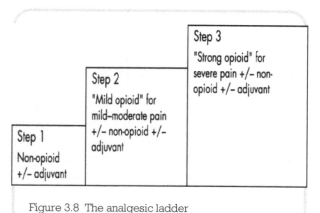

Figure 3.8 The analgesic ladder

Non-steroidal anti-inflammatory drugs

NSAIDs are a group of drugs commonly given to patients who complain of mild to moderate pain.

These drugs are also known to lower the body temperature (they are *antipyretic*) and have anti-inflammatory properties (see Chapter 5). Earlier we discussed tissue injury (see p. 33) and how prostaglandin release is implicated in this. When cells are damaged, they release a substance called *arachidonic acid*. This in turn is utilized in two metabolic pathways, one of these being the cyclo-oxygenase pathway which creates a number of products, among them prostaglandins (we will revisit these pathways in Chapter 5). Prostaglandins, especially the prostaglandin E series, are responsible for making the nociceptors more sensitive. As a result, when pain producing products, such as bradykinins, are released, greater pain is felt by the individual.

NSAIDs are thought to decrease the amount of prostaglandins produced by blocking the cyclo-oxygenase pathway. Hence this group of drugs is effective for a range of conditions, such as pain from arthritis, toothache, periods and even cancer. The blockage of the pathway is useful in terms of the amount of pain we feel; however, it also produces side-effects.

Prostaglandins contribute to our natural balance (homeostasis) and have important roles to play within the body. The prostaglandin E series is responsible for ensuring the mucous lining of our digestive tract remains effective. It also has a role to play in the kidneys, where it helps to maintain the correct pressure for the kidneys to filter water and waste products. Therefore, interference with prostaglandin production has a price and this is shown in the gastrointestinal and renal side-effects of using this group of drugs.

Aspirin

Aspirin was the first drug to be discovered in this category. It has a long history, going back to the fifth century BC and the Greek physician Hippocrates. Aspirin is a weak acid; therefore, it is absorbed better in an acid environment such as the stomach, although the small intestine absorbs the greatest amount of the drug due to its large surface area.

For adults, doses of 300 to 1000mg are generally given four times a day. The correct dose of aspirin naturally depends on the condition being treated. For mild to moderate pain it is usually given at a dose of 300 to 600mg four times a day. Due to its gastrointestinal side-effects, it is best given with or after food in an enteric coated form which discourages breakdown in the stomach and small intestine.

Clinical tip

Aspirin is no longer routinely used with children due to its link with a condition known as Reyes syndrome. This is a rare disorder which affects the liver and central nervous system, usually following an acute viral illness. However, the mortality rate is high at up to 40 per cent.

Other contraindications are also associated with aspirin. The drug should be avoided in patients with known allergies to ibuprofen and naproxen, or with kidney disease, peptic ulcers and gastritis. Patients with a tendency to bleeding disorders (e.g. haemophilia) should also avoid this drug. Taking aspirin with other drugs, such as warfarin (see Chapter 6) is also known to increase the chances of gastrointestinal bleeding. Asthmatic patients should be alerted to the possibility of it causing a severe reaction. It is estimated that one in five patients who suffer from asthma run the risk of having a severe reaction to the drug. Aspirin also

has a number of other side-effects which are dealt with in more detail in Chapter 5.

Ibuprofen

Ibuprofen is another drug that blocks the enzyme that makes prostaglandins, resulting in lower levels of these in the body. Ibuprofen is prescribed for mild to moderate pain, caused by many and diverse conditions. The usual dose for minor aches and pains, including painful periods and a high temperature, is 200 to 400mg every four to six hours.

As with other drugs in this class ibuprofen is usually enteric coated and should be taken with or just following food. The drug does have suspected interactions. If taken with lithium (a mood stabilizer) it may lead to increased levels of lithium due to its influence on lithium excretion by the kidneys. Ibuprofen has a similar effect on an antibiotic known as gentamycin. Gentamycin levels may rise, thus increasing the risk of side-effects. It should also be avoided during pregnancy as no adequate studies have been completed on its safety during this period.

Side-effects are similar to other drugs in this category, such as rash, abdominal pain, nausea, diarrhoea and heartburn (dyspepsia). Renal function is also affected so ibuprofen should be used cautiously in patients who already have a degree of renal impairment or congestive cardiac failure.

Diclofenac

Diclofenac is another NSAID that you will come across on a regular basis. It is frequently prescribed to patients who have pain and inflammation due to rheumatic disease and is often the drug of choice for musculoskeletal pain in the joints, muscles and tendons. It is also becoming increasingly popular as a post-operative analgesic.

Diclofenac comes as an immediate-release tablet, a liquid-filled capsule and an extended-release (long acting) tablet to take by mouth. Some diclofenac tablets have an enteric coating designed to prevent the absorption of the drug in the stomach, and thus reduce the risk of stomach irritation and indigestion.

Clinical tip

Diclofenac dispersible tablets are dissolved in water before taking. The diclofenac solution is rapidly absorbed from the gut, so this type of tablet provides pain relief more quickly than the other types. However, the solution is more likely to irritate the stomach lining, because it doesn't have the advantage of the protective enteric coat. The dispersible tablets are therefore most suitable for short-term use and should not be used for longer than three months.

and use of NSAIDs in these patients should be approached cautiously. Individuals with asthma are more likely to experience allergic reactions to diclofenac and other NSAIDs.

Clinical tip

Sometimes, stomach ulceration and bleeding can occur without any abdominal pain. Black tarry stools (melaena), weakness and dizziness upon standing may be the only signs of internal bleeding. So listen to the patient and monitor them for these signs and symptoms.

Extended release tablets contain a higher dose of diclofenac and are designed to release this slowly and continuously over a few hours. This provides more prolonged pain relief, and these tablets are usually taken once a day, less commonly twice a day.

Diclofenac immediate release tablets and capsules are usually taken two to four times a day. Diclofenac can also be given in suppository form or as a gel which is absorbed by the skin.

Diclofenac should be taken with food to reduce stomach irritation. The recommended dose for most conditions is 100–200mg daily. However, the dosing intervals depend on the formulation used and the condition being treated.

Like other NSAIDs diclofenac is associated with several suspected or probable interactions that affect the action of other drugs. The most common side-effects of diclofenac involve the gastrointestinal system. The drug can cause ulcerations, abdominal burning, pain, cramping, nausea, gastritis and even serious gastrointestinal bleeding and liver toxicity, rash, kidney impairment, ringing in the ears and lightheadedness are also seen. People who are allergic to other NSAIDs should not use diclofenac. NSAIDs reduce the flow of blood to the kidneys and impair their function. The impairment is most likely to occur in patients with already reduced kidney function or congestive heart failure,

As with ibuprofen, diclofenac may increase the blood levels of lithium by reducing the excretion of lithium by the kidneys. Increased levels of lithium may lead to lithium toxicity. This is particularly important to bear in mind if the patient is being treated with lithium for other problems. Diclofenac may also reduce the blood pressure, lowering effects of blood pressure medications. This may occur because prostaglandins play a role in the regulation of blood pressure. Individuals taking oral anticoagulants such as warfarin should avoid diclofenac because it also affects the clotting cascade by its actions on prostaglandins, which in turn could increase the patient's international normalized ratio (INR) (see Chapter 6).

Paracetamol

Paracetamol relieves pain and fever in adults and children and is probably the most widely used medicine in fulfilling this role. It can be prescribed by a doctor or pharmacist, but generally it is bought as an OTC medicine. It is over 100 years since the drug was first discovered and we are still learning what the mechanism of action is.

Paracetamol does not appear to have any significant action on either of the cyclo-oxygenase pathways. This helps to explain why it has freedom from the gastrointestinal side-effects typical of other NSAIDs. A third previously unknown pathway is initiated by an enzyme found in the brain and spinal cord. This enzyme is specifically affected by paracetamol and it is this effect that explains its effectiveness in relieving pain and reducing fever without GI side-effects.

> **Clinical tip**
>
>
>
> The recommended adult dose for paracetamol is 1000mg six hourly, and no more than eight tablets in a 24-hour period. As long as this dose is adhered to, there are no toxic effects. There are no groups of people who should not take paracetamol and interactions with other medicines are rare.

Paracetamol is quickly absorbed by the body and its peak serum levels occur within approximately 30 minutes to two hours after ingestion. Elimination is also rapid: paracetamol has a half life of about two hours. It is vital that the recommended dose be adhered to, because a substantial overdose of paracetamol is likely to result in liver damage and requires immediate treatment. When paracetamol is broken down by the liver it produces an active byproduct. In order to neutralize this, the liver attaches a substance known as glutathione to it. In overdose, the rate of the byproduct increases far quicker than the liver can manufacture glutathione. Eventually the liver stores are exhausted and the reactive byproduct starts to damage the liver tissue itself.

Treatment of overdose requires skilled hospital management. An antidote called n-acelylcysteine is available and is given intravenously. This restores the liver's capacity to produce glutathione and, therefore, protect the liver tissue from damage. It is important that the antidote is administered quickly and it is best given within 12 hours of ingestion. However, it has been shown that even 48 hours post-ingestion the antidote has beneficial effects.

> **Clinical tip**
>
> It is worth remembering that paracetamol is often combined with decongestant ingredients in cold and flu remedies. Therefore, this should be considered by the patient if taking the full dose so that accidental overdose can be avoided. The size of retail packs is also intended to reduce the risk of overdose. Pharmacies are limited to a maximum 32-tablet pack and shops are limited to packs of 16. Multiple packs can be purchased, however, if more than 100 tablets are needed, but a doctor's prescription will be necessary.

Opioid analgesics

These drugs commence where the NSAID group finish. Therefore, they are given for moderate to severe pain (please refer to the WHO analgesic ladder). Opioid drugs are a class of natural, synthetic and semi-synthetic agents and are used for their analgesic, anti-tussive (stop you coughing) and anti-diarrhoeal properties. This class of drug is derived from the opium poppy and its properties have been used for centuries.

> **Clinical tip**
>
>
>
> You may find a number of terms that are used interchangeably when describing drugs in this category: 'narcotic', 'opiate' and 'opioid'.

All opioids exert their effect through binding with specific receptors called opioid receptors located in the central nervous system (brain and spinal cord) or peripherally in the GI tract. There are four types of opioid receptor and they are designated by the Greek letters μ (mu), κ (kappa), σ (sigma) and δ (delta). Different opioid analgesics bind in different ways with a variety of these receptors, so explaining why a range of effects and side-effects can occur.

Opioid drugs are agonistic in nature: they mimic our own endorphins, bringing about a similar analgesic reaction. There are numerous opioid analgesic preparations, some natural (e.g. morphine and codeine) and some synthetic (e.g. diamorphine, methadone, fentanyl and meperidine). We will focus on morphine as a strong agonistic opioid, fentanyl as a synthetic opioid and codeine as a moderate agonist or weak opioid.

Morphine

Opioid drugs are thought to work through a number of mechanisms. You will recall that at the beginning of this chapter we discussed the importance of calcium channels opening in order to bring about the transmission of a nerve signal across a synapse. Morphine is thought to block these channels from opening so that the pain signal breaks down. It is also thought that morphine opens potassium channels in neurones, so making the inside more negative, a condition known as *hyperpolarization*. This makes the firing of a pain neurone more difficult.

The most important effects of morphine occur on the central nervous system and the GI tract and include:

- **Analgesia.** This term refers to the loss or relief of pain but without the loss of consciousness. Morphine is useful in both acute and chronic types of pain. It not only raises the level at which pain is initiated (higher threshold) but also alters the brain's perception of the pain. The person is still aware of the pain but does not recognize it as an unpleasant sensation.
- **Euphoria.** When a person takes morphine it makes them feel a powerful sense of contentment and well-being, often described as a 'rush'. This in itself is a useful effect as pain often leads to anxiety and agitation. Euphoria tends to be present in patients who are prescribed the drug for acute pain, whereas patients with chronic longstanding pain may lose this effect.
- **Respiratory depression.** This is caused by the respiratory centre in the brain stem becom-

ing less sensitive to the respiratory drive of carbon dioxide. It is one of the more troublesome side-effects that you need to be aware of, particularly as it can occur with therapeutic doses. It is the commonest cause of death in acute opioid poisoning.

- **Depression of the cough reflex.** This does not match the analgesic or respiratory depressive effects of morphine. Therefore, weaker opiates, such as codeine, can be used in antitussive preparations.
- **Nausea and vomiting.** This occurs in up to 40 per cent of people who are prescribed morphine when they first start to take the drug. As they become tolerant of the medicine this effect is reduced. These side-effects are thought to be brought about by morphine's effects on a particular area of the brain known as the chemoreceptor trigger zone (CTZ).
- **Pupillary constriction.** 'Pinpoint pupils' are caused by morphine. The drug stimulates a pair of cranial nerves called the occulomotor nerves which cause this phenomenon.
- **Effects on the GI tract.** Morphine reduces the rate at which the GI system moves (motility). This leads to constipation, which is often severe and very troublesome for the patient. All patients receiving morphine should be considered for an aperient. Morphine also affects the smooth muscle of the biliary tract, causing a rise in the pressure within this system. It is due to this effect that morphine should be avoided in people suffering from biliary colic due to gallstones: if morphine is given it might actually increase the pain rather than lessen it. The general slowing of the gut may affect the absorption of other drugs.

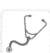

Clinical tip

The discovery of pinpoint pupils is still used as a significant diagnostic feature of opiate overdose as other causes of unconsciousness tend to cause the pupils to dilate.

Despite its side-effects, morphine is still regarded as the gold standard by which other analgesic medications are measured. Absorption of the drug from the GI tract is not particularly good. Significant first pass effect occurs in the liver, and therefore subcutaneous, intramuscular or intravenous injections are usually given.

Repeated doses of morphine cause tolerance, resulting in the need to prescribe a higher dose of the drug to achieve the same effect. Physical and psychological dependence does occur.

Fentanyl

Fentanyl is a powerful synthetic opiate analgesic similar to but approximately 100 times more potent than morphine, with 100mcg of fentanyl approximately equivalent to 10mg of morphine. It is typically used to treat patients with severe pain, or to manage pain after surgery. It is also used to treat people with chronic pain who are physically tolerant to opiates.

Fentanyl is a narcotic analgesic acting predominately at the μ-opiate receptor. Apart from analgesia, the fentanyls as a group produce drowsiness and euphoria, the latter being less pronounced than with morphine. The most common side-effects include nausea, dizziness, vomiting, fatigue, headache, constipation, anaemia and peripheral oedema. Tolerance and dependence develop rapidly after repeated use. Characteristic withdrawal symptoms (sweating, anxiety, diarrhoea, bone pain, abdominal cramps, shivers or 'goose flesh') occur when use is stopped.

Serious interactions can occur when fentanyls are mixed with heroin, cocaine, alcohol and other central nervous system depressants such as benzodiazepines. The use of human immunodeficiency virus (HIV) protease inhibitors such as ritonavir has been reported to increase plasma levels and reduce elimination of co-administered fentanyl. As with morphine, overdose results in respiratory depression which is reversible with naloxone (see p. 46).

As it has a wide range of uses for both acute and chronic pain, fentanyl comes in a number of formulations, including intravenous injection, lozenges and transdermal patches. Such skin patches should only be used to control moderate to severe chronic (around-the-clock, long-lasting) pain that cannot be controlled by the use of other pain medications in people who are tolerant to narcotic pain medications. Fentanyl patches should not be used to treat mild pain, short-term pain, pain after an operation or medical or dental procedure, or pain that can be controlled by medication that is taken as needed. Patches are usually applied to the skin once every 72 hours. The doctor may start the patient on a low dose and gradually increase this, not more often than once every three days at first, and then not more often than once every six days.

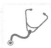

Clinical tip

The medication in fentanyl patches is contained in a gel that is sealed between layers of the patch. If this gel leaks from the patch, remove it immediately without touching the gel. If you do touch the gel, immediately wash the area with large amounts of clean water. Do not use soap, alcohol or other cleansers.

Fentanyl skin patches can be habit forming. The patient should be reminded not to apply more than one patch at a time, nor to wear them for any longer than the period prescribed. Equally they should not cease usage without consulting their doctor, as there is a danger of symptoms of withdrawal such as restlessness, teary eyes, runny nose, yawning, sweating, chills, hair standing on end, muscle aches, large pupils, irritability, anxiety, backache, pain in the joints, weakness, stomach cramps, difficulty falling asleep or staying asleep, nausea, loss of appetite, vomiting, diarrhoea, fast heartbeat and rapid breathing.

Codeine

Codeine is a less potent analgesic than morphine, and is frequently referred to as a weak opioid. However, it has an advantage over morphine in that it is well absorbed when taken orally, although when increased to higher doses for severe pain the analgesic effect does not increase above a certain range. Large amounts of the drug do not provide extra analgesia; therefore, it is only suitable for mild to moderate pain. Codeine has a lower potential for dependency making abuse of the drug less likely, although cases have been reported. The drug has a good anti-tussive quality at doses that do not produce analgesia; therefore, it has the potential for use in cough medicines. However, in most non-prescription cough medicines it has been replaced by newer drugs such as dextromethorphan, a synthetic narcotic, which has the same anti-tussive properties.

Codeine is used in drugs which are classed as *analgesic mixtures*. For example, co-codamol tablets contain codeine phosphate 8mg and paracetamol 500mg. Another example that you may come across regularly is co-dydramol, which contains dihydrocodeine 10mg and paracetamol 500mg per tablet.

Opioid antagonists

As discussed above, respiratory depression is a side-effect of opiates. Therefore, in opioid overdose, an antidote is necessary. This comes in the form of a drug called Naloxone which has great attraction to all three opioid receptors. Naloxone blocks the actions of morphine and our own endorphins by occupying the opioid receptors but not bringing about any response, so effectively stopping anything else connecting to the receptor.

Naloxone therefore quickly reverses the effects of opioid drugs.

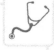

Clinical tip

The main clinical use of Naloxone is to treat respiratory depression caused by opioid drugs in overdose, whether accidental or intentional. It is usually given intravenously and its effects are immediate. It has a relatively short half life as it is quickly metabolised by the liver. Therefore, when treating a patient you may see the drug repeatedly used in order to maintain respiratory function.

Adjuvant drugs

Opioid antagonists are used in combination with non-opioid and opioid drugs to facilitate the management of pain in patients, particularly complicated and chronic pain. They can be divided into two broad categories: co-analgesic drugs and drugs that are used to relieve the side-effects of analgesics.

Co-analgesics include drugs such as antidepressants, anticonvulsants, local anaesthetic agents and anxiolytics. Drugs commonly used to treat side-effects include laxatives, antihistamines, neuroleptics and antiemetics.

Case studies

① Dawn Mason, a 40-year-old woman, has undergone major abdominal surgery. The medical staff have decided to change her analgesia from opioids to non-steroidal anti-inflammatory medication as she is four days post-surgery. A health care assistant approaches you and asks you to explain the mode of action of the different types of analgesia and why the patient is now stepping down from one set of analgesia to another. Discuss this with reference to:

- the mode of action of these two drugs;
- the importance of stepping down post-operative analgesia;
- the maintenance required to achieve a steady plasma concentration of analgesic;
- how you would put this information into terms that the health care assistant will understand.

② Alex Smith is a 9-year-old boy who has sustained a broken arm after falling from his bike. The doctor has prescribed him paracetamol and ibuprofen. The dose he can have for each drug is:

- ibuprofen, 200mg every 6–8 hours;
- paracetamol, 500mg every 4–6 hours, maximum 2g in 24 hours.

You have to explain to Alex and his parents how these drugs work and the importance of regular medication to manage Alex's pain. Discuss this with reference to:

- pharmacodynamics: mode of action of the two drugs;
- pharmacokinetics: the need for regular dosing to achieve therapeutic plasma concentration;
- how you would put this information in terms that Alex and his parents will understand.

Key learning points

Introduction

➢ Pain lets us know about tissue damage.
➢ It is a defence mechanism.
➢ We can suffer pain without tissue damage.
➢ Pain is a difficult concept to define.
➢ At rest the inside of a neurone carries a negative charge.
➢ In order for the neurone to fire the inside must become positive.
➢ Sodium moves into the neurone to make it positively charged.
➢ The pre-synaptic neurone allows calcium to enter.
➢ The neurotransmitter allows the post-synaptic neurone to be excited or inhibited.
➢ Pain is received by nociceptors.
➢ Nociceptors are fired by heat, pressure or chemicals.
➢ Nociceptors are non-adapting, high threshold fibres.
➢ Pain is transmitted by A delta and C fibres.
➢ A delta and C fibres synapse in the dorsal horn of the spinal cord.
➢ The pain impulse is interpreted in a number of areas in the brain.
➢ The analgesic system is a descending one.
➢ It is thought to close the gate to pain stimuli.
➢ Endorphins, dynorphins, enkephalins are important in modifying pain.
➢ Nociceptive pain results from tissue damage.
➢ Neuropathic pain is damage to nerves in the peripheral or central nervous system.

Local anaesthetics

➢ Produce a reversible loss of sensation.
➢ There are two classes: esters group and amides.

→

←

➤ Block sodium channels in the neurone.
➤ Usually presented as dilute preparations (e.g. lignocaine 1 per cent).
➤ Can cause vasodilation (so are often given with adrenaline).
➤ Can be given topically, via infiltration, as a nerve block, as an epidural, as a spinal anaesthetic or as an intravenous injection.
➤ Can cause central nervous and cardiovascular side-effects.

Non-steroidal anti-inflammatory drugs

➤ Used for mild to moderate pain.
➤ Lower body temperature and have anti-inflammatory properties.
➤ Block the production of prostaglandins.
➤ Block cyclo-oxygenase pathways.
➤ Limit prostaglandin E effects on the nociceptors.
➤ Have marked gastrointestinal and renal side-effects.
➤ Paracetamol damages the liver if the recommended dose is not followed.
➤ Paracetamol overdose is treated with n-acetylcysteine.

Opioid analgesics

➤ Given for moderate to severe pain.
➤ Work on receptors in the central nervous system.
➤ Some drugs are natural compounds and some are synthetic agents.
➤ Block entry of calcium into pre-synaptic neurone.
➤ Open potassium channels making it harder for the pain neurone to fire.
➤ Main effects are on the central nervous system and gastrointestinal tract.
➤ Morphine is the gold standard by which other opioids are measured.
➤ Morphine can cause tolerance and dependence.
➤ Fentanyl is a powerful synthetic opiate analgesic similar to but approximately 100 times more potent than morphine.
➤ Fentanyl is used to treat patients with severe pain, or to manage pain after surgery.
➤ Fentanyl is also used to treat people with chronic pain who are physically tolerant to opiates.
➤ Codeine is a weak opioid.
➤ Naloxone is given to reverse the effects of morphine.

Calculations

1 Pethidine 100mg in 2ml is available to you. However, the patient has been prescribed 75mg. How much do you give?

2 A patient requires 1000mg of paracetamol in liquid form. The stock you have contains 100mg in 5ml. How many ml would you give?

3   Codeine is available in three strengths as tablets, 5mg, 10mg and 20mg. What is the least number of tablets you can give if the prescription is a dose of 50mg?

4   13mg of intramuscular morphine is required to be given. You have 5mg in 1ml ampoules. How much would you give?

5   A patient is prescribed an injection of 80mg of Pethidine. You have available 100mg in 1ml. How much fluid would you draw up?

6   You have Pethidine injection 100mg in a 2ml solution. The patient is prescribed 75mg. How much do you draw up?

7   The maximum dose of paracetamol is 4g in a 24-hour period. Tablets are 500mg. What is the maximum number of tablets you can give in a 24-hour period?

8   A patient requires 4mg of intramuscular morphine sulphate. You have reconstituted the morphine to make a dose of 10mg in 1ml. How much do you draw up?

9   35mg of codeine is to be given to a patient subcutaneously. You have available 50mg in 1ml. How much do you administer?

10   Fentanyl 75mcg is to be given intravenously. You have fentanyl 0.1mg in 1ml available. How much would you draw up?

For further assistance with calculations, please see Meriel Hutton's *Essential Calculation Skills for Nurses, Midwives and Healthcare Practitioners* (Open University Press 2009).

Multiple choice questions

Try answering these multiple choice questions to test what you have learned from reading this chapter. You can check your answers on page 198.

1 What is the role of prostaglandins in the reception of pain?

a) They make the nociceptors more sensitive
b) They directly stimulate the nociceptors
c) They stimulate the release of bradykinin
d) They only act on receptors in the central nervous system

2 Local anaesthetic agents work by

a) Opening potassium channels
b) Opening sodium channels
c) Blocking potassium channels
d) Blocking sodium channels

3 Why are some local anaesthetics given with adrenaline?

a) Adrenaline is needed in order for local anaesthetics to work
b) Adrenaline counteracts the vasodilation caused by local anaesthetics
c) Adrenaline makes local anaesthetics work more quickly
d) Adrenaline helps the local anaesthetic enter the cells

→

←

4 NSAIDs work by

a) Blocking production of bradykinin
b) Making the neurone fire more frequently
c) Stimulating the body's own analgesic system
d) Blocking production of prostaglandins

5 Why is it important to tell a patient who has been prescribed paracetamol to be careful when buying OTC medicines?

a) It could be expensive for them
b) You must only take paracetamol on its own
c) Paracetamol is often combined with cold and flu remedies
d) Paracetamol easily interacts with OTCs

6 Ibuprofen must be taken with caution if the patient is also taking lithium: why?

a) The patient may forget to take the medicine
b) It may increase the lithium level in the blood
c) It will make the lithium inactive
d) Ibuprofen also affects mood

7 One of the mechanisms of opiates is thought to be

a) Blockage of calcium channels
b) Opening of calcium channels
c) Blockage of sodium channels
d) Opening of sodium channels

8 Which of the following is *not* a receptor for morphine?

a) Mu
b) Kappa
c) Epsilon
d) Delta

9 Why is it good practice to ensure patients are prescribed an aperient when taking morphine?

a) Because morphine makes some people vomit
b) The patient will be having a poor diet
c) The patient is not likely to be moving
d) It reduces the rate at which the gastrointestinal system moves

10 What drug is given to reverse the effects of morphine?

a) Neomycin

b) Nandrolone

c) Naloxone

d) Neostigmine

Recommended further reading

Beckwith, S. and Franklin, P. (2007) *Oxford Handbook of Nurse Prescribing*. Oxford: Oxford University Press.

Brenner, G.M. and Stevens, C.W. (2006) *Pharmacology*, 2nd edn. Philadelphia, PA: Saunders Elsevier.

Clayton, B.D. (2009) *Basic Pharmacology for Nurses*, 15th edn. St Louis, MO: Mosby Elsevier.

Coben, D. and Atere-Roberts, E. (2005) *Calculations for Nursing and Healthcare*, 2nd edn. Basingstoke: Palgrave Macmillan.

Cornock, M. (2005) Pain relief and the law, *Nursing Standard*, 19(51): 28.

Downie, G., Mackenzie, J. and Williams, A. (2007) *Pharmacology and Medicines Management for Nurses*, 4th edn. Edinburgh: Churchill Livingstone.

Gatford, J.D. and Phillips, N. (2006) *Nursing Calculations*, 7th edn. Edinburgh: Churchill Livingstone Elsevier.

Godfrey, H. (2005) Physiology of pain: understanding pain, part 1: physiology of pain, *British Journal of Nursing*, 14(16): 846–52.

Godfrey, H. (2005) Pain management: understanding pain, part 2: pain management, *British Journal of Nursing*, 14(17): 904–9.

Karch, A.M. (2008) *Focus on Nursing Pharmacology*, 4th edn. Philadelphia, PA: Lippincott Williams & Wilkins.

Lapham, R. and Agar, H. (2003) *Drug Calculations for Nurses: A Step-by-step Approach*, 2nd edn. London: Arnold.

Mann, E. and Redwood, S. (2000) Improving pain management: breaking down the invisible barrier, *British Journal of Nursing*, 9(19): 2067–72.

Melzack, R., and Wall, P.D. (1965) Pain mechanisms: a new theory. *Science* 150: 971–979.

National Institute for Health and Clinical Excellence (NICE) (2007) *Clinical Guideline 52: Drug Misuse – Opioid Detoxification*. London: NICE.

Simonson, T., Aarbakke, J., Kay, I., Coleman, I., Sinnott, P. and Lyssa, R. (2006) *Illustrated Pharmacology for Nurses*. London: Hodder Arnold.

Trounce, J. (2000) *Clinical Pharmacology for Nurses*, 16th edn. New York: Churchill Livingstone.

WHO (World Health Organization) (1966) *Cancer Pain Relief*. Geneva: WHO.

4

Antimicrobials

Chapter contents

Learning objectives
Introduction
  Bacterial infection
Interference with folate
  Trimethoprim
Beta-lactam antibiotics
  Penicillins
  Cephalosporins
  Clavulanic acid
Interference with protein synthesis
  Tetracyclines
  Chloramphenicol
  Aminoglycosides
  Macrolides
  Lincosamides
Inhibition of bacterial DNA
  Fluoroquinolones
Antibiotic resistance
  Causes of antibiotic resistance
Issues with neonates and children
Drugs used to treat tuberculosis
  Isoniazid
  Rifampicin
  Pyrazinamide
Viral disease
  Viral mechanisms
Human immunodeficiency virus
  Antiretroviral therapy
  Nucleoside reverse transcriptase
    inhibitors
  Non-nucleoside reverse transcriptase inhibitors
  Protease inhibitors

Other antiviral drugs
  Aciclovir
  Ganciclovir
  Amantadine
  Immunoglobulins
  Interferons
Fungal infections
  Moulds
  True yeasts
  Yeast-like fungi
Antifungal drugs
  Amphotericin
  Nystatin
  Griseofulvin
  Azoles
    Ketoconazole
    Fluconazole
    Miconazole
  Flucystosine
  Terbinafine
  Future antifungal therapy
Protozoa
  Apicomplexa
    Quinine
  Flagellates
    Metronidazole
  Amoeboflagellates
    Tinidazole
Case studies
Key learning points
Calculations
Multiple choice questions
Recommended further reading

Learning objectives

After studying this chapter you should be able to:

- Describe a bacterial cell.
- Explain the mode of action of a range of antibiotics used in practice settings.
- Demonstrate an understanding of what unwanted effects antibiotics have on humans.
- Discuss drugs that are used to treat tuberculosis.
- Define what is meant by viral disease.
- Describe the mode of action and side-effects of antiviral medicines.
- Identify the three main causes of fungal infection.
- Explain how antifungal medicines act.
- Demonstrate an understanding of the links between the pharmacology of antimicrobial therapies and the care given by the health practitioner.
- Correctly solve a number of drug calculations with regard to antimicrobial medicines.

Introduction

Infectious disease is a major cause of death and disability throughout the world. Many micro-organisms live either inside or on the outside of the human body. These cause disease only when our resistance is lowered through other diseases or when our natural barriers have been affected by disease or trauma. Other micro-organisms are present in the external environment and are taken into our bodies through eating and drinking, breathing or on physical contact.

Micro-organisms that live in or on our bodies for the most part have a harmless relationship with us and can be beneficial – for example, bacteria in the GI system break down foodstuffs allowing us to absorb vitamin K. Unfortunately, at times of vulnerability these same organisms can cause infection and damage. Many other micro-organisms not normally present in the body attempt to invade our tissues, causing damage which can be life-threatening. Any invasion or abnormal growth pattern of micro-organisms which causes our body to defend itself is an *infection*. An example would be peritonitis – the inflammation of the delicate serous membrane which lines the abdominal and pelvic cavities and covers the organs which lie within.

Infectious micro-organisms are categorized into four main groups: bacteria, viruses, protozoa and fungi. Bacteria and fungi are capable of existing independently of their host – i.e. us. Some protozoa and certainly viruses need the mechanisms from our cells in order to replicate and grow. A further category of infectious agent is called a *prion*. These have been particularly press-worthy over the years as they cause bovine spongioform encephalopathy (BSE).

This chapter is designed to give you an introduction to some of the medicines used in combating infections caused by micro-organisms. Drugs used to combat the variety of micro-organisms which may cause us harm are referred to as *antimicrobials*. The chapter is in no way comprehensive and is intended to whet your appetite to read further, so increasing your knowledge. The chapter covers antibiotic therapy, antiviral therapy, antiprotoza therapy and finally antifungal therapy. We have tried to give examples of common drugs that you may come across in practice rather than concentrate on a range of drugs that you may only encounter rarely.

Bacterial infection

We are surrounded by bacteria, most of which are harmless. Having said this, it is probably safe to say that more deaths and disease have been caused by bacteria than any other cause.

Bacteria are classified into a number of types based on how they appear through a microscope – i.e. the shape of them. Some look like rods, and are called *bacilli*. Some are round in shape and are called *cocci*. Others have a spiral or corkscrew shape and are known as *spirochaetes*. Bacteria are also categorized by whether they take up a stain called *gram stain*. Bacteria that absorb this stain are termed *gram positive*, while those that do not are *gram negative*.

The reason for the difference in the uptake of gram stain is a difference in the cell walls of the bacteria. Gram positive bacteria have a simple cell wall whereas the cell wall of gram negative organisms is much more complex. Difficulty in penetrating this complex wall is likely to be why some antibiotics are less effective against gram negative than gram positive bacteria.

Bacteria cells are different from those of humans. Bacteria do not have a nucleus and so are called *prokaryotes*. Our cells do have a nucleus and are called *eukaryotes*. This and other differences between bacteria and human cells is important as antibiotics are designed to target these differences, thus destroying the bacteria while leaving our own cells intact.

On the very outside of a bacterium is a wall made largely from a sugar called peptidoglycan. This is unique to prokaryotic cells. Beneath this wall is a plasma membrane very similar to our own and consisting of a sandwich of phospholipids and proteins. The cell wall and plasma membrane together are called the *bacterial envelope*.

A bacterium contains cytoplasm which carries similar organelles to our own. However the genetic material is arranged in one long strand that floats around in the cytoplasm. A prokaryotic cell does not have any mitochondria and energy production is carried out in the plasma membrane (see Figure 4.1).

Antibiotics are often described as being *bactericidal*: in other words, they kill bacteria, usually very rapidly. They are also *bacteriostatic*, which means that the antibiotic prevents the growth of an infection but does not eradicate it totally. Instead it gives the body's natural defence mechanisms time to recognize and deal with the infection. The distinction between these two terms is not black and white because in certain conditions a bactericidal antibiotic may only have a bacteriostatic effect and vice versa. Their effects are somewhat governed by dosage, outside influences and the health of the patient.

Selective toxicity is the ability of the antimicrobial to harm a pathogen (bacteria) without harming our own cells. Therefore, when discussing selective toxicity in terms of an antibiotic, health care practitioners are referring to the range between the dose necessary to inhibit or destroy the bacteria and the dose at which our own cells become harmed. Thus an antibiotic that is far more toxic to the bacteria than our cells is said to have a greater selective toxicity.

Interference with folate

Folate is a vitamin required by both bacterial and human cells. Human cells have evolved a mechanism to directly take up folate from the interstitial fluid. Bacteria on the other hand have to make their own folate and cannot absorb it directly from the environment.

A group of antibiotics called sulfonamides exploit this difference between bacterial and mammalian cells. Bacteria need a substance called PABA (see Chapter 3) in order to make the folate they need. Sulfonamides fool the bacteria into taking up a substance that looks identical to PABA but cannot be used by the bacteria. In this way, they prevent the cell reproducing and are therefore bacteriostatic in nature.

Trimethoprim

This sulfonamide drug is sometimes given as a combination called co-trimoxazole. Trimethoprim is given orally as it is well absorbed by the GI system. The drug is usually given to treat urinary and respiratory infections and may be prescribed with sulfamethoxazole as co-trimoxazole. However, this tends to be limited to treating patients with acquired immuno-deficiency syndrome (AIDS) for a particular type of pneumonia.

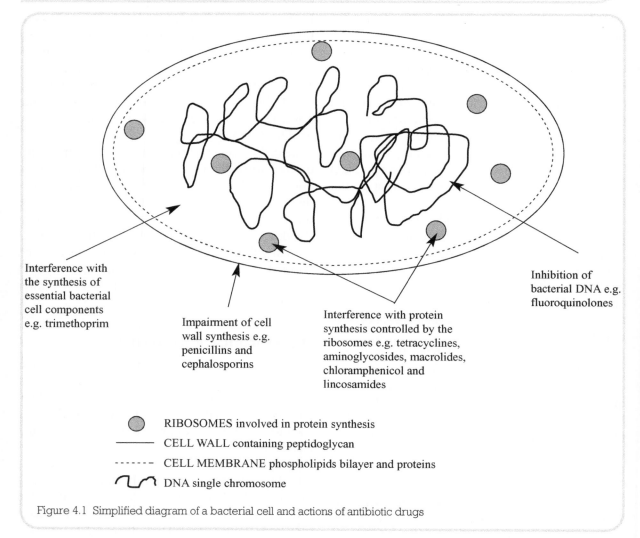

Interference with
the synthesis of
essential bacterial
cell components
e.g. trimethoprim

Impairment of cell
wall synthesis e.g.
penicillins and
cephalosporins

Interference with protein
synthesis controlled by the
ribosomes e.g. tetracyclines,
aminoglycosides, macrolides,
chloramphenicol and
lincosamides

Inhibition of
bacterial DNA e.g.
fluoroquinolones

RIBOSOMES involved in protein synthesis

CELL WALL containing peptidoglycan

CELL MEMBRANE phospholipids bilayer and proteins

DNA single chromosome

Figure 4.1 Simplified diagram of a bacterial cell and actions of antibiotic drugs

The side-effects of trimethoprim include nausea, vomiting, certain blood disorders and skin rashes. The drug can also lead to the development of a type of anaemia due to its affects on folate. This is usually counteracted by giving the patient folinic acid.

Beta-lactam antibiotics

Peptidoglycan makes up to 50 per cent of the cell wall in bacteria. In some cells this wall is very thick. However, certain antibiotics stop the bacterial cell from making this substance, thus rendering the cell useless. This is how drugs such as penicillins and cephalosporins work.

Penicillins

The first penicillin was the naturally occurring benzylpenicillin, and is still used today. The main drawback with this drug is that it is poorly absorbed from the GI tract so can only be administered by injection. Also, due to the length of time it has been used, many bacteria have developed enzyme systems to combat its effects. Therefore, various semi-synthetic versions have been prepared by altering the basic biochemistry of the drug. You will no doubt come across many of these in your experiences within health care settings. Examples include flucloxacillin, ampicillin and amoxicillin. The *-illin* suffix is a useful way of identifying these types of drugs. They can be given orally in a number of forms (tablet, syrup and suspension).

Clinical tip

Pencillin drugs are fairly free from side-effects. The main problem is with hypersensitivity, which is why you must always ask the patient if they have any allergy to penicillin. This information must be documented on the prescription chart and in the nursing records. Skin rashes and fever are common contraindications; much more serious is acute anaphylactic shock.

Penicillins are the drugs most likely to cause anaphylactic reactions, and are thought to be responsible for 75 per cent of anaphylactic deaths. It is sometimes feasible to carry out a skin test for hypersensivity. However the results are not always conclusive and the patient may suffer a severe reaction to only a small amount of the drug. Cefuroxime appears to be a safe alternative but not 100 per cent safe, so care must be taken.

Penicillins can have an adverse effect on the normal bacteria that live in our digestive systems. Sometimes this results in diarrhoea which can lead to a lack of vitamin K absorption. In addition, infections by micro-organisms not sensitive to penicillin can take place. In other words, the fine balance in the digestive system between good and bad bacteria can be altered by penicillin therapy.

Cephalosporins

These drugs are chemically related to the penicillin group. Similarly, many semi-synthetic drugs have also been developed. As a result there is a large range of medicines in this group that can be prescribed for infections.

These drugs work in the same way as penicillin in that they affect the production of the peptidoglycan wall of the bacterium. Today they are extremely important, due to the production of enzymes against the biochemical make-up of penicillins which have made those drugs less effective in preventing infection.

Some cephalosporins may be given orally; for example, cefalexin. However, most of this group of drugs are given via the IV or SC routes; for example, cefuroxime and cefotaxime are administered in this way. After being absorbed, cephalosporins are widely distributed in the tissues of the body. Some can actually cross over the BBB; for example, cefuroxime. This drug therefore is useful for infections in the central nervous system. Excretion is mainly by the kidneys but some cephalosporins, for example, cefoperazone, are eliminated in the bile. These drugs can work on both gram negative and gram positive bacteria but this depends on which drug is prescribed.

Side-effects are similar to those of the penicillin group, so hypersensitivity reactions can occur. Between 0.5 and 6.5 per cent of penicillin-sensitive patients will also be allergic to cephalosporins, so it is essential to check for any documentation of allergies when assessing the patient. Diarrhoea is also a significant side-effect with this group of medicines.

Clavulanic acid

Clavulanic acid is a beta-lactamase inhibitor. Beta-lactamases are enzymes that are produced by some bacteria and are responsible for their resistance to beta-lactam antibiotics like penicillins (cephalosporins are relatively resistant to beta-lactamase). These antibiotics have a common element in their molecular structure: a four-atom ring known as a beta-lactam. The lactamase enzyme breaks the ring open, deactivating the molecule's antibacterial properties.

Clavulanic acid itself has only a weak antimicrobial activity, despite sharing the β-lactam ring that is characteristic of beta-lactam antibiotics.

However, when combined with a penicillin group antibiotic it gives the potential to overcome certain types of antibiotic resistance including resistance in bacteria that secrete beta-lactamase, and which otherwise would inactivate most penicillins. In its most common form, the potassium salt potassium clavulanate is combined with amoxicillin (co-amoxiclav, commercially known as Augmentin). Despite this, some bacterial strains have emerged that are resistant even to such combinations.

The use of clavulanic acid with penicillins is not risk-free however, and there has been an associated increased incidence of cholestatic jaundice and acute hepatitis during therapy or shortly after – in particular in men and those over the age of 65. The associated jaundice is usually self-limiting and very rarely fatal.

The UK Committee on Safety of Medicines (CSM) recommends that amoxicillin/clavulanic acid preparations be reserved for bacterial infections likely to be caused by amoxicillin-resistant β-lactamase-producing strains, and that treatment should not normally exceed 14 days.

Interference with protein synthesis

Protein synthesis takes place in the ribosomes. However, ribosomes are different in eukaryotes (i.e. our cells) than in prokaryotes (i.e. bacterial cells). This is another difference that can be exploited by antibiotic therapy.

Tetracyclines

This group of drugs acts by stopping bacterial cells from making essential proteins. The group includes tetracycline, oxytetracycline and minocycline. The spectrum of these medicines is wide and they are effective against both gram negative and gram positive bacteria.

Tetracyclines are usually given by mouth but can be administered by other routes. Absorption is better if they are given on an empty stomach as they can be absorbed erratically and this is not helped by the presence of food.

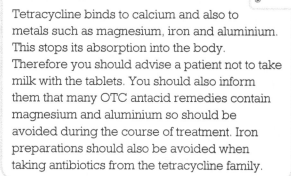

Clinical tip

Tetracycline binds to calcium and also to metals such as magnesium, iron and aluminium. This stops its absorption into the body. Therefore you should advise a patient not to take milk with the tablets. You should also inform them that many OTC antacid remedies contain magnesium and aluminium so should be avoided during the course of treatment. Iron preparations should also be avoided when taking antibiotics from the tetracycline family.

GI problems are probably the most common unwanted effect from this group of antibiotics. This is usually due to direct irritation by the medicine and also a decrease in the balance of normal intestinal bacteria (flora). Because they bind calcium, it is possible for tetracycline drugs to be deposited in growing bones and teeth. This can cause staining of teeth, underdevelopment of the teeth (hypoplasia) and bone deformities. For these reasons tetracyclines should not be given to children, pregnant women or nursing mothers.

As with other antibiotics many strains of micro-organisms have now developed resistance to this group, therefore making them less useful in clinical practice.

Chloramphenicol

This antibiotic is similar in action to the tetracycline group. It is a broad spectrum antibiotic which can be used against gram positive and gram negative organisms. It is rapidly and completely absorbed when given orally and reaches its maximum effect in the plasma in two hours. If necessary it can be given by other routes – for example, topically into the eye for conjunctivitis. The drug has a wide distribution in the tissues of the body including the cerebrospinal fluid, around the brain and spinal cord.

The most important unwanted effect of this drug is that it causes a severe depression of the bone marrow. This results in a fall in all blood cell elements. This side-effect is rare but can occur in low doses in some individuals. Chloramphenicol should only be given to babies with extreme caution as they do not have the capacity to metabolize and excrete the drug. This may result in a combination of signs and symptoms called 'grey baby syndrome' in which the baby vomits, has diarrhoea, is flaccid, has a low temperature and is ashen grey in colour. This syndrome carries a high mortality rate of 40 per cent. However the drug is given for certain acute or serious infections, for example gram negative bacteria which cause meningitis.

Aminoglycosides

This group of antibiotics includes gentamycin, streptomycin, tobramycin and neomycin and acts by inhibiting bacterial protein synthesis. Aminoglycosides are useful against both gram negative and gram positive organisms. However, these drugs are only bacteriacidal in the presence of oxygen. Therefore, bacteria that thrive in oxygen-poor environments (anaerobes) are only minimally affected. As with other groups the resistance of micro-organisms to these drugs is increasing all the time.

One of the most common drugs in this group is gentamycin. This is given by either the IV or IM route as it is not absorbed by the GI system. The drug has a fairly rapid half life of two to three hours, necessitating the dose being given three times daily. The main problem with this drug is its serious toxic effects. It can have a devastating effect on the apparatus in the inner ear (ototoxicity). This means that the patient may suffer damage to either their hearing or their ability to balance. The second major side-effect is damage to the kidney tubules (nephrotoxicity). This can be reversed if the drug is stopped.

Due to these major problems it is important that gentamycin is kept within a therapeutic range in the plasma. The plasma level half an hour following injection should be between 5 and 10mg per litre and the level just prior to injection should be 2mg per litre.

> **Clinical tip**
>
> The side-effects of gentamycin mean that gentamycin levels must be monitored by medical staff. A blood sample is usually taken at specific times – either just prior to administration or half an hour afterwards. It is therefore very important that doctors have this information relayed to them accurately by the nursing staff.

Macrolides

Erythromycin was the only drug in this group for many years. However, several new drugs have been developed that you may come across – for example, clarithromycin and azithromycin. As with the other antibiotics in this section macrolides inhibit protein synthesis in the bacterium.

Erythromycin destroys a similar range of micro-organisms as penicillin and is the first drug of choice if a patient has a penicillin allergy. The drug is mainly prescribed for gram positive organisms and spirochaetes. It has very limited success with gram negative organisms.

All drugs in this group can be given orally and they spread throughout most tissues of the body. They do not cross the BBB into the central nervous system and they do not penetrate synovial fluid. Macrolides possess different half lives which is why some are given more often in a day than others. They have an unusual action in that they are taken up and concentrated in phagocytic cells – the group of white cells responsible for digesting bacteria. Inside these phagocytic cells there are pockets of cell-destroying enzymes called lysosomes. Macrolides are absorbed into these pockets and therefore considerably enhance the phagocytic killing capacity of these cells.

Unwanted GI problems are the main issue when taking these medicines. If erythromycin is administered intravenously rather than orally, a degree of inflammation and damage to the vessel that the drug is entering (thrombophlebitis) can be expected.

Clinical tip

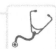

It is important that you monitor the intravenous site regularly for pain, swelling and redness. If this is present medical staff should be informed and you should document the condition of the intravenous site in the nursing care plan. Medical staff may discontinue the intravenous therapy until they have recannulated the patient.

Lincosamides

The drug of note in this group is called clindamycin. Its mechanism of action involves inhibition of protein synthesis in bacteria. It works against a range of organisms which include gram positive cocci and a range of anaerobic bacteria.

The drug can be given orally or by other routes and becomes well distributed in the body tissues, including bone. Like a number of other antibiotics it does not have the capacity to cross the BBB. The usual dose is 150mg four times daily.

Unwanted effects are mainly GI in nature and the patient may suffer from diarrhoea. In rare cases this may become life-threatening as they develop a condition called *pseudomembranous colitis*. This is an acute inflammation of the colon caused by toxins released from micro-organisms that are resistant to clindamycin; an example would be infection with a bacteria called *clostridium difficile*.

Inhibition of bacterial DNA

You will be aware from your non-stop reading of anatomy and physiology texts that DNA stands for deoxyribonucleic acid, which is found in all living cells and carries the organism's genetic information. In bacteria this information is what we call *supercoiled*. Some writers have likened this to putting 15 metres of cotton material into a matchbox. In order for the bacteria to survive through replication this information needs to be copied. To do this an enzyme is needed to uncoil parts of the supercoiled material. The enzyme that brings this about in the bacterial cell is called *topoisomerase II*. A group of antibiotics called fluoroquinolones affect the ability of the bacteria to use topoisomerase II.

Fluoroquinolones

The most common antibiotic in this group is called ciprofloxacin, which is a *broad spectrum* antibiotic. It is useful as it is effective against micro-organisms that have become resistant to penicillins, cephalosporins and aminoglycosides. This drug can be given orally and is well absorbed. It enters many tissues and particularly concentrates in the kidneys, prostate gland and lungs, making it ideal for fighting infection in these areas of the body.

Clinical tip

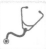

As with tetracyclines the rate of absorption of fluoroquinolones is diminished by metals such as aluminium and magnesium, so they should not be used while taking antacids that contain these elements.

Unwanted effects are not frequent, usually mild in nature and disappear rapidly once the drugs have been stopped. In the main, GI problems like diarrhoea are reported. Sometimes people also complain of developing a skin rash, headaches and dizziness. One of the main interactions with this drug develops if it is given to asthmatic patients who are receiving a drug called theophylline. The ciprofloxacin inhibits enzymes in the liver that are normally responsible for the metabolism of theophylline. This results in a build up of theophylline in the plasma, eventually reaching toxic proportions.

Clinical tip

Ciprofloxacin should not be used for patients taking theophylline. If there is no alternative the doctor should closely monitor levels of theophylline in the blood if they have no alternative but to give theophylline.

Antibiotic resistance

One of the foremost concerns in modern medicine is *antibiotic resistance*. Simply put, if an antibiotic is used long enough, bacteria will emerge that cannot be killed by that antibiotic. Infections exist today that are caused by bacteria resistant to some antibiotics, and existence of antibiotic-resistant bacteria creates the danger of life-threatening infections that don't respond to antibiotic treatment.

There is an alarming rise in the occurrence of antimicrobial resistance. For example, *Staphylococcus aureus* is a prevalent bacterium carried by humans that can cause a number of problems, from mild skin infections to serious diseases including food poisoning, wound infections, pneumonia and toxic shock syndrome. In 2002, the WHO reported that more than 95 per cent of this bacterium worldwide is resistant to penicillin, and 60 per cent to its derivative methicillin.

Causes of antibiotic resistance

Misuse of antibiotics occurs in medicine, agriculture and household products. Common examples include erroneous antibiotic prescriptions for non-bacterial infections and the addition of antibiotics to livestock feed and cleaning agents, which have helped create a reservoir of antibiotic-resistant bacteria.

Sometimes irregular combinations of bacteria have perpetuated drug-resistant microbes. One example was when *staphylococcus aureus* was shown to develop vancomycin resistance genes through cohabitation with the vancomycin-resistant bacteria, *enterococcus faecalis*, in the wound of a hospitalized patient. Through mechanisms of genetic exchange between bacterial species, the mere coexistence of these two particular bacteria helped to bring about drug resistance in the *staphylococcus aureus*.

Enhanced transmission of resistance factors, or the increased efficiency with which resistance genes are exchanged, is another important way that antibiotic resistance is perpetuated. Factors that contribute to enhanced transmission include the survival of patients with chronic disease, an increased number of immunosuppressed individuals, substandard hospital hygiene, more international travel and budget cuts in health care administration.

Profit also has a role to play in the development of drug resistance. The pharmaceutical industry has increasingly been busy with hugely profitable 'blockbuster' drugs for allergies and depression, and 'lifestyle' drugs for conditions such as baldness and impotence. This has led to decreased antibiotic and vaccine research and development.

In many cases, drug-resistant bacteria have been met with antibiotics that are nothing more than replicas of earlier drugs. There is an urgent need for new avenues of therapeutic treatment, and a new era of prophalytic (preventative) treatment has now begun.

Issues with neonates and children

Antibiotic misuse is most likely to occur in children with ear infections (otitis media), the number one reason a child is brought to a doctor. Antibiotic therapy is the most common treatment of ear infections, with amoxicillin being the first choice. The side-effects of amoxicillin include upset stomach, diarrhoea, allergic reactions and nappy rash.

Research suggests that when antibiotics are used at the beginning of an ear infection, the frequency of recurrence may be almost three times greater than if antibiotics are delayed or not used (AHRQ 2000). Antibiotics do not just go after the pathogenic or 'bad' bacteria. They also destroy the beneficial bacteria necessary and vital to good health. Among the more important beneficial bacteria are *lactobacillus acidophilus* and *bifidobacterium bifidus*. They help protect the body against infection. Depleting these organisms can disrupt the balance of the body and lead to increased susceptibility to infection by fungi, bacteria, viruses and parasites. Additionally, when antibiotics are used excessively, depleting the beneficial bacteria, there may be an overgrowth of yeast in the body. This may lead to candida infection (thrush).

Children are growing and therefore require adequate nutrition; however, antibiotics adversely affect many nutrients, particularly those needed by the immune system to fight infection, such as vitamins A and C. One of the most common side-effects of antibiotics is diarrhoea. This causes a loss of nutrients, especially magnesium and zinc, which are important in growth and repair.

Sweeteners, dyes, flavourings and other additives are found in antibiotics prescribed to children. These may include saccharin, sucrose and red dye. Some dyes may be reactive with medicines such as aspirin and paracetamol, which are commonly given to a child during an illness. Even tiny amounts of the chemical additives in antibiotics can cause an allergic reaction in a sensitive child.

Drugs used to treat tuberculosis

Despite hopes that tuberculosis (TB) might be eradicated from the UK, in recent years there has been an increase of the disease in this country and it is not uncommon to be nursing someone suffering from TB.

TB is usually caused by inhaling the *mycobacterium tuberculosis* organism. This bacteria has a very tough envelope and can survive for long periods in dry conditions. This coating also protects the organism, making it resistant to destruction by the body's natural defences. The bacterium can invade and survive within our phagocytic cells. The damage to our tissues is usually due to the body's inflammatory response to the infection rather than the result of any toxin released by the organism.

Initial infection of the lungs is called *primary TB*. The bacteria is engulfed by phagocytic cells in our lungs. These cells attempt to communicate with T lymphocytes which attempt to resist the infection but the increase in phagocytic cells at the site of infection is relatively ineffective. Instead, more and more of the phagocytic cells become infected by the bacteria and are carried into the lymphatic system where they eventually reach what is known as the *hilar lymph nodes* within the lungs.

The body manages to 'wall off' these infected phagocytes by creating pockets which are known as *tubercles*. These are balls of infection with a necrotic (dead) centre surrounded by infected phagocytic cells wrapped in a capsule of collagen (protein) fibres. These tubercles may then remain in the lungs but the patient suffers no further symptoms of the disease.

The tubercles are now little time bombs ready to explode. If the person's immune system becomes compromised the condition is activated again from its dormant state. Reactivation may take place under a number of circumstances – for example, poor nutrition, the age of the patient and lowered immune system.

This reactivation is called *secondary TB*. The lung tissue itself now becomes necrotic, creating large cavities. As with the tubercles, these cavities remain encapsulated by connective tissue and may lie dormant or become reactivated once again.

Miliary TB is a condition in which the patient cannot make an adequate response to the initial infection. This leads to weight loss, extreme tiredness (lethargy) and coughing. The organism is now invading the blood and sets up camp in a variety of tissues including the lungs, meninges, spleen, liver and bone marrow. If this is not treated, death ensues. It is with this in mind that we will now look at the treatment of TB. First line drugs will be discussed and include isoniazid, rifampicin and pyrazinamide.

Isoniazid

This drug is specific against mycobacteria and is therefore very helpful in the treatment of TB. It is bacteriostatic when the organisms are not active, but becomes bacteriocidal when they start to divide and multiply. The drug diffuses through cells and crosses the BBB into the cerebrospinal fluid. This point is important as it penetrates well into the tubercles described earlier.

The normal dose for an adult is up to 300mg per day and is usually given as a tablet. Some people break down this drug rapidly in the liver and some do not. The latter group tend to have a better therapeutic response as the drug manages to reach a more constant level in the plasma.

Side-effects are related to the dose given, the commonest being skin problems. Patients who metabolize isoniazid more slowly are more at risk of side-effects if they are dosed too often. Isoniazid affects enzymes in the liver that break down certain anti-convulsant drugs. Phenytoin, ethosuximide and carbamazepine can all be increased in the plasma if given with isoniazid.

Rifampicin

Rifampicin acts by interfering with a substance called ribonucleic acid (RNA) in the bacteria so affecting protein synthesis within the organism. This antibiotic has a broad range of activities and is effective against both gram positive and gram negative organisms. It is the most active agent in the fight against TB to date. It has the ability to get right inside the phagocytic cells that have ingested the tubercle bacillus. Once inside, it can destroy the tubercle bacillus at will.

The drug is well absorbed by the GI system and therefore is given in tablet form, usually in a dose of between 450 and 600mg daily prior to eating breakfast. It is able to gain entry to a wide group of tissues and fluids.

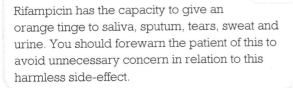

Clinical tip

Rifampicin has the capacity to give an orange tinge to saliva, sputum, tears, sweat and urine. You should forewarn the patient of this to avoid unnecessary concern in relation to this harmless side-effect.

Unwanted effects are not common. Some patients may suffer skin problems, a raised temperature and GI upsets such as nausea and diarrhoea. Liver damage, with a yellow discoloration of the skin (jaundice), whites of the eyes (sclerae) and mucous membranes has been reported and can prove fatal.

Clinical tip

Because of the risk of liver damage patients who are prescribed rifampicin should have their liver enzymes tested prior to commencing the therapy.

As with isoniazid, rifampicin affects enzymes in the liver that help to break down certain drugs.

Rather than inhibiting the pathways, rifampicin induces them. In other words, drugs such as warfarin, glucocorticoids, opiates, oral hypoglycaemic agents and oestrogen are all broken down more rapidly. This means dosing needs to be adjusted accordingly.

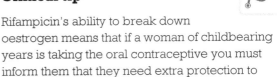

Clinical tip

Rifampicin's ability to break down oestrogen means that if a woman of childbearing years is taking the oral contraceptive you must inform them that they need extra protection to avoid pregnancy.

Finally, you will find that rifampicin is often given alongside other antibiotics to combat TB. This is in order that we do not give the organism the opportunity to develop resistance. As this is the most active treatment the last thing we want to do is render it useless.

Pyrazinamide

Pyrazinamide is well absorbed orally and becomes widely distributed in the tissues and fluids of the body. It penetrates well into the meninges so is particularly useful if the disease spreads into this area.

Pyrazinamide works in a similar way to rifampicin in that it gains entry to the phagocytes that have ingested the bacteria and destroys it. Side-effects include the raising of plasma uric acid levels, so causing gout. GI symptoms and a raised temperature have also been reported. Liver failure is also a possibility especially if the drug is given in high doses. However, high doses are uncommon as a combination of drugs is the preferred technique in treating the organism (see above). Liver function tests should, however be carried out prior to drug commencement.

Viral disease

Viruses are very different from bacteria. They are a lot smaller and essentially have a core of either DNA or RNA surrounded by a coat of protein (capsid). The coat plus its contents are referred to as the *nucleocapsid*. Some viruses are even more protected in that they have developed a further coat of phospholipids from the host cell (the cell in which virus lives), and some of the viruses own glycoproteins.

At some point in their lifetime, everyone in the world will have been infected by a virus. Conditions such as chickenpox, shingles, conjunctivitis, warts, measles, mumps and rubella are all caused by viral infections.

Viral mechanisms

A virus is basically a type of parasite that gets into a cell and then uses the cell's machinery for its own purposes. Viruses do not have the ability to reproduce and replicate themselves so they have to borrow these mechanisms from their host cell. Certain viruses also carry the mechanisms to reproduce (replicate) inside the host cell without using the host cell's machinery to help them. This particle of potential infection is called a *virion*.

The virus gains access to the cell by locking onto a receptor that carries out some normal activity. The virus is then taken into the interior of the cell by a process of *endocytosis*. Basically, the cell swallows the infective virus and allows it to enter the cytoplasm. Once inside the host cell the nucleic acid centre of the virus starts to use the host cell's machinery to help it replicate more of its kind (viral replication). This can take various forms depending on the type of virus.

Some viruses are called DNA viruses. This means that they replicate by latching into and becoming part of the host cell's DNA. Once they have achieved this they can direct the manufacture of more viruses. Other viruses are called RNA viruses and use the host's RNA, linking with the viral RNA code so that the cell manufactures the proteins that go into building new viruses within the cell. Finally, *retroviruses* work by copying a viral blueprint onto a piece of DNA. This viral DNA is then linked into the host's DNA and so the host starts creating new viruses as part of its normal activity.

Compared to bacterial treatment with antibiotics it is very difficult to produce antiviral drugs because viruses live within our own cells. Once inside, they can also switch off mechanisms for their detection, along with the self-destruct mechanisms that our cells contain. This leads to a very slippery customer indeed when trying to develop treatment. A further problem in dealing with viruses is that by the time the body has recognized it has been invaded, a large amount of the virus has been manufactured.

Human immunodeficiency virus

This virus causes acquired AIDS, which is a growing problem in some parts of the world. The worst affected area is sub-Saharan Africa. In the UK in the 1980s the number of people with HIV diminished, some argue due to large television campaigns informing the population about the disease. However, the incidence levels in many sexually transmitted diseases (STDs) including HIV and AIDS are on the increase, in particular with men and women in the older age range.

HIV is the result of the invasion of a particular lymphocyte called a *helper T cell* (T4 cells). These cells are very important in defending the body and are linked to the immune response. Once the person has been infected with the virus it can be transmitted to other people in a variety of ways: through sexual intercourse, blood or transplanted organs and tissues, from an infected mother to her foetus and by breastfeeding.

HIV may remain dormant within the body for many years and most people are quite unaware that they have contracted the disease. However, it is possible by blood testing to confirm within a few weeks of infection whether the person has acquired the virus. The time taken for this ticking bomb to explode in terms of loss of immune response in the individual varies from months to years. An average time from diagnosis of HIV to death from AIDS is about two years in an untreated patient.

The virus targets cells with certain receptors on their surface. Examples of these cellular 'name badges' are CD4 and CCR5. The virus attaches itself to receptors on these cells and is taken in. Once inside it works on the principles of a retrovirus. In other words, it produces its own DNA by using a viral enzyme and then embeds the viral DNA into the host's DNA. The host cell then begins to make proteins which will be made into new viruses. These will then eventually leave the cell and gain access to cells of their own by recognizing the 'name badges' on them. As the cells divide the integrated viral DNA also divides and becomes part of the new cell. This is called *proviral DNA*. It effectively means that any helper T cell on division passes on the ability of the daughter cells to produce more viruses.

Antiretroviral therapy

Antiviral therapy is aimed at using a combination of agents that act at different points in the replication of the virus within the human cell. One of the main reasons for using a combination of drugs is to delay the onset of resistance in any one of the therapies. Currently, antiviral drugs used in the treatment of AIDS fall into two broad categories: *reverse transcriptase inhibitors* and *protease inhibitors*. We will now focus on each of these drug classes.

Nucleoside reverse transcriptase inhibitors

Reverse transcription is the second phase in the HIV life cycle. HIV genes are carried on two strands of RNA; however, in order to enter the nucleus of a human cell the virus must change the genetic code into a strand of DNA. It does this by using a viral enzyme called *reverse transcriptase*. Nucleoside reverse transcriptase inhibitors are designed to block the action of reverse transcriptase.

Some examples of drugs from this class are zidovudine, abacavir and lamividine. All may be given orally but there are some differences in the frequency of administration. Zidovudine and abacavir have short half lives and lamividine has a long half life which affects dosing. All these drugs diffuse through a range of tissues, however, zidovudine achieves the best concentration in the cerebrospinal fluid, about 65 per cent of that which it achieves in the plasma.

Adverse reactions to this family of drugs are not pleasant. Zidovudine can cause bone marrow depression leaving the patient open to all types of infection. Abacavir may cause hypersensitivity reactions including rashes and high temperatures. Lamividine in comparison has only mild side-effects such as headaches and some GI symptoms.

Non-nucleoside reverse transcriptase inhibitors

These drugs have the same effect as the nucleoside reverse transcriptase inhibitors but have a different method of achieving the response. Quite often, you will find both types of drugs being given alongside each other. There are two main drugs in this family: nevirapine and efavirenz.

Both are given orally. Nevirapine is 100 per cent bioavailable compared to efavirenz which is between 50 and 60 per cent bioavailable. The half lives of nevirapine and efavirenz, compared with their relatives, are considerably longer. Both drugs have elimination half lives of between 30 and 40 hours.

The main adverse affect of nevirapine is the development of a rash. This occurs in up to 20 per cent of patients taking the drug. Other common side-effects are headaches, a high temperature and lethargy. Efavirenz has similar problems in that about 25 per cent of people taking it will develop a rash. This drug may also lead to disorientation and lack of concentration.

Protease inhibitors

If the viral RNA manages to make a copy of its genetic blueprint onto DNA, then this is carried into the nucleus of the human cell. Here, another viral enzyme called *integrase* joins the viral DNA onto the human DNA, and hides it. Then, when the cell tries to make new proteins, it also makes new viral proteins. A new class of drugs is currently being developed that will be aimed at blocking the actions of integrase.

Eventually, these proteins are assembled into new HIVs in the endoplasmic reticulum and golgi apparatus of the cell. This assembly-line relies on an enzyme called *protease* to cut the proteins into either functional units of the virus or viral enzymes.

Protease inhibitors block this stage of viral replication in the cell. Examples of current

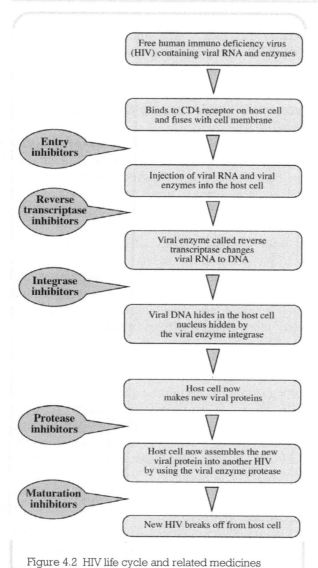

Figure 4.2 HIV life cycle and related medicines

sugar levels and hyperlipidaemia. These symptoms are not good news if you happen to be diabetic and have HIV.

All the drugs in this family also cause enzyme inhibition, especially to pathways which break down benzodiazepines. Therefore, the concentration of these drugs will rise if given together with protease inhibitors.

The combination of drugs now given for HIV has dramatically improved the prognosis (see Figure 4.2). This has obviously had a lessening effect on AIDS cases and deaths in industrialized countries. However, as noted above, in many developing countries cases of both disease processes continue to rise in number.

Other antiviral drugs

Aciclovir

You might have come across this drug and used it yourself. The trade name is Zovirax and if you suffer from cold sores you have probably used the product. The drug is used for a number of viral infections including conjunctivitis, genital warts and shingles. Rarely, it can be used in treating acute chickenpox and encephalitis in immunocompromised patients.

Aciclovir works by stopping the herpes virus from reproducing and infecting further cells of the body. The drug becomes more active once it has entered the cell that is infected by the virus. The herpes virus works as a DNA virus and aciclovir acts by blocking an enzyme called *DNA polymerase*. The virus needs this enzyme to copy its genetic code from a strand of RNA to a strand of DNA. This process is necessary for the virus to multiply and continue to infect its host. By blocking the action of DNA polymerase, the drug prevents the host cell making copies of the virus. This controls the virus and buys the immune system time to deal with the initial infection.

Aciclovir can be given orally, intravenously or topically (e.g. cream). If a patient is prescribed the drug in dispersible form they should be encouraged to take the tablet dissolved in a full glass of water.

protease inhibitors are saquinavir and indinavir (there are six inhibitors currently available in the UK). All these drugs are given orally, however saquinavir is subject to metabolic breakdown by an extensive first pass effect. In terms of distribution, cerebrospinal fluid levels are very low with saquinavir whereas with indinavir they rise to 76 per cent of that which the drug achieves in the plasma.

All these drugs cause GI disorders and endocrine disturbances such as insulin resistance, high blood

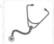

Clinical tip

It is good practice to advise patients to drink plenty of water when taking aciclovir orally to avoid over-concentration of the drug (six to eight pints of water per day). It is also advisable to tell the patient to take the whole course of treatment and if they miss a dose to take the next one but not to double up on the tablets if they forget a dose.

Common drug reactions occur in just over 1 per cent of patients taking the medication. These include nausea, vomiting, diarrhoea and sometimes headache. In high doses the drug may cause hallucinations.

Clinical tip

When aciclovir is administered by the IV route you should observe and document any changes at the site of the IV therapy. This is important because if the drug enters the tissues rather than going into the vein it may cause local pain and irritation. As a cream aciclovir can cause some dryness and flaking of the skin and, in some cases, redness. When applied to the eye the patient should be warned that it may cause a short-lasting stinging sensation.

Aciclovir should not be given in pregnancy as it could cause chromosomal mutations to occur. This is because the foetal cells are dividing rapidly and the tissues are becoming specialized.

Ganciclovir

This drug also stops the virus passing on its genetic code from a piece of RNA to a piece of DNA. However, it targets a different type of virus, the *cytomegalo* virus. Infection by this virus in people with an intact immune system is usually mild. Therefore this drug is used only in people whose immune systems are not fully functional (they are

Clinical tip

The reason for problems in transplantation stem from the fact that the person's immune system has to be switched off. This is in order that the body does not recognize the transplanted tissue as foreign and therefore is prevented from attacking it.

Ganciclovir is given intravenously and is not rapidly broken down in the cells like aciclovir. It has been shown to remain in infected host cells for as long as 20 hours. However, its side-effects are serious. The medicine causes bone marrow depression leading to depletion in white cells and platelets. This usually recovers once the treatment has stopped. It is also possible that the drug may be carcinogenic and it is therefore only used to fight life- or sight-threatening disease.

Amantadine

This drug is active against the influenza A virus but not the B virus. It works by stopping the virus gaining entry to the host cell and also by stopping any newly made viruses from leaving the cell after replication. Amantadine is well absorbed orally and so is usually given in tablet form in a dose of up to 200mg daily. Unwanted effects are rare and occur in only 5 to 10 per cent of patients. They include dizziness, insomnia and slurred speech.

Immunoglobulins

Immunoglobins contain antibodies against specific viruses that the patient may encounter in the population. These antibodies set to work on the viral envelope and attempt to destroy it. They also prevent virus attachment to host human cells. If used before the onset of disease immunoglobulins can be protective to the body.

Interferons

Interferons are a group of proteins that are made by our cells in order to help combat invasion by viruses. These substances have been commercially developed and are given to help us combat infection.

Interferons are not just one substance but a range of proteins with different properties. Some have antiviral properties, particularly interferon alpha and beta. These medicines work by influencing the ribosome in the cell to stop making the viral proteins. In this way they stop the virus from replicating.

These medicines reach optimum capacity in the plasma after five hours but do not cross over the BBB. Interferon alpha may be used in the treatment of hepatitis B and AIDS-related kaposi sarcoma, as well as for hepatitis C.

Side-effects are common and include the development of a high temperature (fever), headaches and pain in the muscles (myalgeia). If the therapy has to be repeated, more serious side-effects can occur such as bone marrow depression, the development of rashes and dramatic hair loss (alopecia).

Fungal infections

Fungi exist in our environment and on our skin (known as *commensals*). As with bacteria most fungi are not pathogenic unless the immune system becomes depleted. Fungi can invade superficial tissues but more serious damage, sometimes life-threatening, comes from the invasion of deeper tissues.

It is somewhat ironic that the reason for a significant upturn in fungal infections has been due to the widespread use of broad spectrum antibiotics, which have decreased the populations of bacteria that normally compete with fungi, therefore allowing the fungi to flourish unchecked. A further reason for the increase in the number of fungal infections is disease processes such as AIDS and the use of more immunosuppressant drugs and cancer therapies. There are three types of fungal organism that are capable of causing disease in the human body and these are discussed below.

Moulds

These grow as long strands which are called filaments. They then begin to intertwine with each other. These intertwined moulds are referred to as *mycelium*. Examples of moulds which can become infective are the dermatophytes and aspergillus. A typical condition caused by infection with dermatophytes (dermatomycoses) is tinea (ringworm). This can affect the scalp (tinea capitus), the groin (tinea cruris) and the body (tinea corporis). The athlete's foot (tinea pedis) fungus belongs to this group of fungi.

A more serious condition caused by moulds is aspergillus – a serious lung infection. It can become problematic in patients having bone marrow transplants and is a leading cause of death in this group of individuals. Another group at risk of developing this condition are immunocompromised patients. Aspergillus causes an allergic reaction in the tissues of the lung. This leads to thrombosis and necrosis of the lung tissues as the pulmonary blood vessels become subject to invasion by the fungus.

True yeasts

These are unicellular and have either a round or oval shape. Yeasts, known as *cryptococcus neoformans* can lead to serious meningitis or endocarditis. Again these mainly occur in individuals whose immune systems have been compromised in some way. This organism is common in soil, especially where there are bird droppings. Infection quite often arises after a person has inhaled the fungi.

Yeast-like fungi

These look like yeasts but under certain conditions develop filaments. The most frequent is called *candida albicans*. This lives quite happily as a commensal organism in our GI system and in the vagina.

> ### Clinical tip
>
>
>
> Candida albicans becomes problematic (pathogenic) when people become stressed, are immunocompromised or when they are taking courses of antibiotics. At such times they may develop oral thrush or vaginitis.

More serious illnesses can occur that can cause inflammation of the lining of the heart (endocarditis) and in some cases these fungi can have fatal consequences – for example in cases of septicaemia.

Antifungal drugs

Most fungal infections are superficial, however they can become systemic (widespread) in immunocompromised patients. Amphotericin has for many years been the first line antifungal agent, though several other drugs have been developed. This section will focus on two main treatment groups: antifungal antibiotics and synthetic antifungal agents.

Amphotericin

This drug was first used over 50 years ago and is a macrolide antibiotic (which means it inhibits protein synthesis in the bacterial cell) and is very complex in its biochemical structure.

Amphotericin works by targeting fungi and some protozoa. This specificity is thought to occur as the drug likes a substance called ergosterol. Ergosterol is the main lipid in the membrane of a fungus as opposed to our cells, in which the main lipid is cholesterol. Once the drug has adhered to the membrane of the fungi it starts to punch holes

in it, so causing it to lose potassium. Potassium is the major intracellular positively charged ion (cation) and its loss will lead to the death of the organism.

Amphotericin is poorly absorbed from the GI system and so the oral route of administration is only used when the patient has a fungal infection of this system. It can be given topically.

> ### Clinical tip
>
>
>
> For systemic infections amphotericin needs to be given by slow IV infusion. This method has serious side-effects, for example nephrotoxicity. It also depletes the body of potassium and magnesium. The liver may become impaired in its function, and a low platelet count (thrombocytopenia) and severe anaphylactic reactions are also common. The drug is also irritant to the lining of the blood vessels, hence thrombophlebitis during and following IV administration is necessary.

Due to the unwanted effects of amphotericin researchers have been working hard to come up with other ways of administering this drug. One reasonably promising development has been to deliver it in little spheres of lipid so that it is in a protected form until it binds with the fungal membrane. Amphotericin is mainly used for serious and life-threatening fungal infections because of its serious side-effects.

Nystatin

This is an antibiotic that disrupts the membrane of the fungus. It is very poorly absorbed from the GI system and so its use is limited to fungal infections of the GI tract – for example, oral thrush.

Nystatin can also be effective against candidal infections of the vagina and penis. Administration into the vagina as a pessary every day for 14 days is an effective treatment. Nystatin cream should be applied to the glans penis three times a day for a similar period of time.

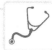

Clinical tip

With oral thrush, nystatin can be given as a liquid preparation or via pastilles that the patient can suck. Oral hygiene and assessment of the mouth is an important aspect of nursing. It is recommended that an oral assessment tool is used. Patients at risk of developing oral candidiasis are those being treated with antibiotics and steroids and it is important that when applying nystatin orally to these individuals you are aware whether they have dentures. If they do, you should soak them in 1 per cent sodium hypochlorite solution overnight and rinse them well before reinserting.

Griseofulvin

Griseofulvin only has a narrow range of activity, which limits its use. The drug is fungistatic and achieves this by stopping the fungus from dividing.

It can be useful in treating dermatophyte infections of the skin and nails due to its ability to be taken up by the basal cells in the epidermis and concentrated in the substance keratin. Keratin is what makes up your nails and is introduced to your skin cells before you shed them.

Griseofulvin is administered orally and its peak plasma concentration occurs after five hours. It has a long elimination half life of approximately 24 hours and causes enzyme induction in the liver; therefore it can affect the metabolism of other drugs the patient may be taking. Side-effects are rare but the drug can cause GI upsets as well as headaches and photosensivity. Treatment needs to continue over a prolonged period of time to prove effective.

Azoles

This group of drugs is manufactured synthetically. Azoles are fungistatic in nature and have a broad spectrum of activity. The mode of action is complex and not fully understood. However, what we do know is that they interfere with a fungal enzyme called P450. This prevents lanosterol from converting to ergosterol, therefore affecting the nature of the fungal membrane and its ability to replicate.

One of the disadvantages of using this group of drugs is that human beings carry cytochrome P450. As a result, some members of the azole group of drugs can also affect the human cytochrome P450 pathways.

Ketoconazole

This is one of the first of this group of drugs to be given orally in order to treat systemic (generalized) fungal infections. It is well absorbed by the body and disperses widely in human tissues and fluid. However, it does not reach therapeutic levels in the cerebrospinal fluid.

The main drawback of ketoconazole is liver damage. This is fortunately rare but can be fatal. Other problems that can result from taking this medication are itching of the skin, GI disturbances and inhibition of adrenocorticoids and testosterone.

Fluconazole

This medication is often advertised on television in connection with preventing vaginal thrush. An oral dose of 150mg is often adequate when treating vaginal candidiasis. Side-effects are generally mild: nausea, abdominal pain and headaches are commonplace. However, although rare, liver disturbances such as hepatitis can occur.

Miconazole

This drug can be given in a number of different ways including orally for GI infections and as a pessary to treat vaginal candidiasis. It can also be purchased as a gel for the treatment of oropharyngeal candidiasis or as a cream for treating lesions of the skin such as dermatophytoses.

As with fluconazole, the side-effects when taken orally are mild with GI disturbance, itching, low blood sodium (hyponatraemia) and other blood disorders being reported.

Clinical tip

More problems arise if miconazole is given by IV infusion and you should be alert to irritant reactions at the site of infusion.

Flucystosine

This is a synthetic antifungal agent that can be given orally. It has a narrow scope of activity and is therefore usually given in combination with other antifungal drugs such as amphotericin.

Flucystosine acts on the fungal DNA. Mutations can occur rapidly and as a result the drug is never given alone as resistance would ensue predictably and rapidly. The drug can also be given by IV infusion and is widely distributed throughout the body. Most of it is excreted in an unchanged form by the kidneys, therefore the dose must be lowered if given to an individual with impaired renal function.

Box 4.1 Administration of antifungal medicines

Route of administration and type	Name of medicine	Uses and side-effects
TOPICALLY		
Creams	Clotrimazole and miconazole	These are used to treat infections of the skin and vagina. These products usually cause no side-effects. Some men and women may develop a mild irritation when applying them to the vagina or penis. Sometimes the antifungal cream is combined with a mild steroid preparation (e.g. hydrocortisone)
Shampoos	Ketaconazole	Used to treat infections of the scalp. No side-effects of note
ORALLY		
Liquids and lozenges	Amphotericin and nystatin	Used to treat candidal infections of the mouth and throat. No side-effects of note
Tablets	Terbinafine and fluconazole	Terbinafine is used to treat nail infections. Fluconazole is used to treat vaginal candidiasis. Usually no side-effects are reported. Can be bought over the counter
INJECTION	Amphotericin and flucytosine	Used to treat serious fungal infection within the body. Risk of serious side-effects. However, these risks must be balanced against the seriousness of the condition

Terbinafine

This drug is given orally for tinea infections of the skin and nails. It is especially useful for these problems as the drug concentrates itself in keratin which makes up the nail tissue and infuses cells in the epidermis.

It can also be locally (topically) applied and penetrates the skin and mucous membranes effectively. Side-effects are limited and only occur in approximately 10 per cent of all patients. Gastrointestinal disturbances, itching, headaches and muscle pains have been reported.

Future antifungal therapy

Resistance to antifungal drugs is now emerging. Fluconazole, for example, has now developed a resistant strain. This occurs especially after long-term use. A particular fungus called *candida krusei* is not sensitive to fluconazole. As a result, a new breed of azoles is now being developed as are drugs which act on fungal protein synthesis and it is almost certain that you will be dealing with medicines in the treatment of fungal infections which have not been mentioned in this chapter.

Protozoa

Protozoa are simple eukaryotic organisms which are made up of a single cell ('protozoa' literally means 'first animal'). These cells have the ability to reproduce through sexual and asexual means. Some protozoa form protective cysts that are capable of withstanding harsh environmental conditions.

Protozoa are often classified by their structure and ability to move. Sporozoa generally produce little movement and invade human cells. Examples of this type of parasite are the plasmodium species which can cause conditions such as malaria.

Some protozoal cells move by wafting an extension called a flagella, rather like using an oar to paddle a boat. This species of protozoa is responsible for diseases such as sleeping sickness and certain forms of vaginitis and urethritis.

Finally, amoebae move by extending parts of their cytoplasm into false limbs called pseudopo-

dia. These organisms are causative agents of dysentery, an acute infection of the intestines, which may spread to other organs, for example, the liver.

This section will briefly outline some of the most common protozoal infections. Antiprotozoal medicines used to treat each of these specific infections will be addressed as we go along. The section is by no means comprehensive and further reading will be necessary in order for you to gain more detailed knowledge.

Apicomplexa

All members of this family of protozoa are parasitic – in other words they invade and use our cells as hosts. They do not have any visible forms of movement and as a result most of them become intracellular in nature. These organisms have complex life cycles involving sexual and asexual reproduction.

The condition known as malaria is caused by this group of protozoa. Malaria is carried by the female mosquito and remains a major cause of death and disability worldwide, causing on average 3 million deaths per year.

The symptoms of malaria include a high temperature (fever), shivering, pain in the joints, headache, vomiting, generalized convulsions and finally coma. These symptoms do not become apparent on initial infection, but usually occur between seven and nine days after the host has been bitten by the mosquito. There are four species of protozoa that are capable of causing malaria.

The bite of an infected female mosquito injects the protozoa into the bloodstream. Within a few minutes the organisms have found their way to the liver. The protozoa mature here over a period of 10 to 14 days. Indeed it is estimated that one species, *plasmodium vivax*, is capable of producing 250 million maturing protozoa from the liver cells in a 14-day period.

After this period the organisms burst out of the liver cells and re-enter the bloodstream. Here they encounter and invade the red blood cells (erythrocytes) and further their development. Once the red blood cell has burst and given up the fully developed protozoa, these are then free to seek out new red cells to infect. This is how the infection escalates rapidly in the body.

Clinical tip

The periodic fever associated with malaria is due to the intermittent bursting of the erythrocytes. On rupturing, the cells not only release their deadly cargo of parasites but also a chemical which affects the temperature-regulating centre in the hypothalamus.

Quinine

We have chosen this drug as it was the first effective treatment of malaria and you will probably be familiar with it. It is derived from the natural world, being synthesized from the bark of the cinchona tree. Quinine is effective against the erythrocytic forms of all protozoa which cause malaria. It has no effect against the development of the protozoa in the liver cells.

The drug works by stopping the protozoa using the proteins from the red cells. Haemoglobin, which is contained in the red cells, is toxic to the parasite. The organism has developed ways in which to render the toxic effects of haemoglobin harmless but quinine interferes with the detoxifying machinery of the protozoa, therefore leading to the death of the organism.

Due to the resistance built up by protozoa to quinine, it is now used only against the plasmodium *falciparum* species. The drug is usually given orally in a seven-day course of treatment. It can however be given via the IV route if the patient is very ill.

Clinical tip

Quinine has a depressant effect on cardiac muscle, so therefore cannot be given as a large one-off dose (bolus). When taken orally it has a very bitter taste which can be problematic as some patients decide not to take the medicine resulting in poor concordance.

In addition to the depressant effect noted above, the drug also has other troublesome side-effects such as diarrhoea and vomiting. If the dose is increased it can lead to dizziness, ringing in the ears (tinnitus), headaches and blurred vision. If the plasma levels rise still further the patient may develop low blood pressure (hypotension), disturbances of heart rhythm (dysrhythmias) and severe central nervous system problems such as coma.

Flagellates

As the names implies, this group of protozoa have flagella which allow them to move. *Trichomonas vaginalis* is a common sexually transmitted organism causing infection in both males and females, although symptoms are more common in women. This disease currently occurs in an estimated 7.4 million new cases each year in both sexes.

The parasite is sexually transmitted through the penis to the vagina during intercourse or by vulva to vulva contact with an infected partner. Therefore, women can acquire the disease from infected men and women, whereas men usually only contract it from infected women.

Most men do not present many signs and symptoms. Occasionally, they may develop a temporary itch inside the penis, a mild discharge or burning on urinating. Women on the other hand develop a frothy green/yellow vaginal discharge which has a strong odour. They may also complain of pain during intercourse and on urinating. Irritation and itching of the vulva are also indications of infection.

Clinical tip

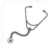

Symptoms do not appear straightaway and usually develop between 5 and 28 days post-exposure.

Metronidazole

This drug interferes with the DNA of the protozoa so destroying its ability to reproduce. It is usually given orally and is rapidly absorbed giving peak plasma levels at between one and three hours. The drug is also available in rectal and intravenous preparations. For use against trichomoniasis it is usually given as a single oral dose.

This drug does not have many unwanted effects. The patient should be warned that they may experience a metallic taste when taking the tablet. Minor GI and central nervous symptoms have been reported.

Clinical tip

The patient should also be informed that metronidazole interferes with the metabolism of alcohol within the body, thus alcohol should be avoided when taking the medication otherwise the patient may have a severe reaction.
When treating trichomoniasis it must also be remembered that in infected men the symptoms may disappear without treatment. This does *not* mean that the protozoal infection has disappeared, and the male is still capable of infecting a woman. As a result both partners should be treated at the same time in order to eliminate the organism. Patients being treated should be advised not to have sex until they and their sexual partner completes the treatment and is symptom-free.
Both parties should also be informed that because they have been treated once does not mean that they cannot become reinfected. Therefore they should be alert to any signs and symptoms of reoccurence.

Amoeboflagellates

These organisms use pseudopodia or flagella in order to aid their movement. *Entamoeba histolytica* is the cause of amoebic dysentery, an infection of the GI system. This species of protozoa is found in contaminated food or drink. *Entamoeba histolytica* infection is potentially life-threatening as the protozoa is able to not only take up residence in the bowel but has the ability to access the bloodstream and therefore infect other organs such as the liver, lungs and brain.

When the amoeba infects the person, the wall of the large intestine is damaged, so causing ulceration and bleeding. Sometimes the person may complain of abdominal cramps (colic), and pain on passing faeces. Bloody, slimy and foul-smelling diarrhoea is also indicative of this infection. The picture for the individual gets much worse if the amoeba breaks through the lining of the gut and invades the peritoneum, causing peritonitis.

The amoeba can now be transported to other organs in the body giving rise to a high temperature and serious consequences. It is possible for the amoeba to create large cysts in the liver and other organs.

Clinical tip

As the main route of entry for the protozoa into the body is via the mouth the best way to avoid infection from amoeboflagellates is by ensuring that anything which is eaten is washed or sterilized properly. Fortunately this disease does not normally occur in the UK and is usually acquired in tropical countries on holiday.

Tinidazole

This drug may be used in combination with metronidazole and diloxanide to treat amoebic dysentery. The drug is given orally as a suspension or tablet. It is usually taken with food as a single dose or once a day for between three and five days. The patient should be encouraged to take the full course even if they feel better. The side-effects are similar to those caused when taking metronidazole.

Clinical tip

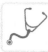

As with metronidazole patients should not consume alcohol when taking tinidazole. Alcohol may cause the patient to have an upset stomach and suffer from vomiting, stomach cramps (colic) and sweating.

Case studies

① Cynthia Day is a 60-year-old woman who has been admitted with a respiratory tract infection. She has been a heavy smoker for 35 years and has been suffering from flu-like symptoms for the past 10 days. On admission, she is pyrexial and dehydrated, although she is able to eat and drink small quantities. Clarithromycin 550mg BD is commenced orally for seven days.

- With reference to the anatomy of a bacterium, explain the mechanism of action of clarithromycin.
- Explain the possible reasons why this antibacterial agent is prescribed in favour of alternatives.
- Explain the clinical observations which you would need to conduct for the duration of Cynthia's treatment.

② Ella Jackson is 18 months old and suffering from an ear infection. The doctor has diagnosed a viral infection and has refused to prescribe antibiotics. Ella's mother does not understand the reason for this and has asked for an explanation. You can reassure her by explaining the difference between viral and bacterial infection. Discuss this with reference to:

- Bacterial and viral infections.
- Mechanism of action of antibiotics.
- Alternative medications to relieve Ella's symptoms of pain and fever.

Key learning points

Introduction

➢ Infectious diseases are grouped into bacterial, viral, fungal and protozoal.
➢ Bacteria are classified as bacilli, cocci or spirochetes.
➢ Bacteria are classified as being gram negative or gram positive.
➢ Antibiotics can be described as being bacteriostatic or bacteriacidal.

Interference with folate

➢ Bacteria need folate to survive.
➢ Trimethoprim is an antibiotic that stops bacteria using folate.

Beta-lactam antibiotics

➢ Stop the bacteria making a robust cell wall.
➢ Examples include penicillins and cephalosporins.
➢ Need to check for allergies before giving these medicines.

Interference with protein synthesis

➢ Tetracycline and chloramphenicol work in this way.
➢ Tetracyclines bind to metals (e.g. magnesium), so are not given alongside antacid preparations.

←

> Aminoglycosides (e.g. gentamycin) require regular blood measurement.
> Macrolides (e.g. erythromycin) can be used in patients allergic to penicillin.
> These drugs cause vomiting and diarrhoea.

Inhibition of bacterial DNA

> Ciprofloxacin performs this function.
> This drug also binds to metals so is not given alongside antacids.

Antibiotic resistance

> Misuse of antibiotics occurs in medicine, agriculture and household products.
> Combinations of bacteria have perpetuated drug-resistant microbes and increased efficiency with which resistance genes are exchanged.
> A lack of economic incentive which led to decreased antibiotic research and development.

Issues with neonates and children

> Antibiotic misuse is most likely to occur in children with ear infections.
> Antibiotics also destroy the beneficial bacteria necessary and vital to good health.
> Antibiotics adversely affect many nutrients.
> Chemical additives in antibiotics can cause an allergic reaction in a sensitive child.

Drugs used to treat tuberculosis

> TB is on the increase.
> Initial infection of the lungs is called primary TB.
> Miliary TB occurs when the person cannot fight the initial infection.
> Isoniazid, rifampicin and pyrazinimide are the main antibiotics used in treating TB.
> Isoniazid causes enzyme inhibition in the liver.
> Rifampicin can cause orange discoloration of saliva, tears and sweat.
> Drugs in this category are often used in combination.

Viral disease

> Viruses are essentially DNA or RNA surrounded by a protein capsule.
> Viruses invade host cells where they use the cell's functions.
> Treating viral disease is more difficult than treating bacterial disease.
> Types of virus include DNA, RNA and retrovirus.

Human immunodeficiency virus

> This is a global problem.
> The virus attacks T helper cells (T4 cells).
> The T helper cells display codes which the virus recognizes.
> HIV is caused by a retrovirus.
> Therapy involves using a combination of drugs.

→

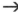

Nucleoside reverse transcriptase inhibitors

➢ Stop the virus using an enzyme called reverse transcriptase.
➢ Zidovudine and abacavir are examples.

Non-nucleoside reverse transcriptase inhibitors

➢ Have the same mode of action as the nucleoside drugs.
➢ Nevarapine is an example.
➢ Nevarapine can cause a rash and fever.
➢ Protease inhibitors stop the virus making new viral proteins in the host cell.
➢ Saquinavir is an example.
➢ Drugs in this group can cause enzyme inhibition in the liver.

Other antiviral drugs

➢ Aciclovir is used to treat cold sores and genital herpes.
➢ Works particularly on DNA viruses by blocking an enzyme called DNA polymerase.
➢ Patient should drink plenty of water when taking the medication.
➢ If administered via IV you need to monitor the site.
➢ Ganciclovir works on DNA virus by blocking enzyme called DNA polymerase.
➢ Used in patients who are immunocompromised.
➢ Causes bone marrow depression.
➢ Amantadine is used against influenza A virus.
➢ Immunoglobins are antibodies against specific viruses.
➢ Interferon stops viruses replicating in host cells by interfering with ribosomes.

Fungal infections

➢ Caused by moulds, true yeasts and yeast-like fungi.

Antifungal drugs

➢ Amphoteracin is a type of macrolide antibiotic.
➢ It targets substance called ergosterol.
➢ It cannot be given orally.
➢ When given intravenously has serious side-effects.
➢ Nystatin disrupts membranes of the fungus.
➢ Used in candidal infections.
➢ Griseofulvin has a narrow range of activity.
➢ Used to treat fungal infection of the nails and skin.
➢ Azoles are synthetically manufactured.
➢ Azoles interfere with fungal P450.
➢ Examples are ketoconazole and fluconazole.
➢ These are both given orally to treat systemic fungal infections.
➢ Flucystosine is another synthetic antifungal drug.

→

←

➤ It has a narrow scope of activity.
➤ It acts on fungal DNA.
➤ Terbinafine is given for tinea infections of the skin and nails.

Protozoa

➤ These are simple eukaryotic organisms.
➤ They are classified into apicomplexa, flagellates and amoeboflagellates.
➤ Apicomplexa cause malaria.
➤ Quinine is given to treat malaria.
➤ Flagellates cause trichomonas vaginalis.
➤ Metronidazole is used to treat trichomonas vaginalis.
➤ Amoeboflagellates cause entamoeba histolytica.
➤ Tinidazole is used alongside metronidazole to treat entamoeba histolytica.

Calculations

1   A doctor has prescribed 800mg of erythromycin. You have 500mg in 10ml suspension. How much suspension would you give?

2   What volume is required for the injection if a patient is prescribed 500mg of capreomycin and all you have in stock is 300mg in 1ml?

3   A patient is prescribed 1000mg of chloramphenicol. The stock on hand contains 250mg in 10ml suspension. How much would you administer?

4   You are required to give a dose of an antibiotic in tablet form. The tablets are available in 25mg. The doctor has prescribed 0.05g. How many tablets do you give?

5   A child weighs 12kg and is prescribed an antibiotic at 15mg per kg. If your stock strength is 200mg in 5ml, what volume would you give?

6   A patient has received a prescription for erythromycin 250mg tablets. How many tablets are required to complete their seven-day course of 500mg four times a day?

7   Your patient weighs 95kg. How much gentamycin (80mg/2ml), should you give for a dose of 5mg per kg (maximum 400mg)?

8   You have a bottle of amoxicillin syrup containing 250mg in 5ml. How much do you need to give 100mg?

9   You have a vial of gentamycin containing 80mg in 2ml. How much do you need to administer 300mg?

10   You need to give 1g of erythromycin orally. You have erythromycin suspension 250mg in 5ml. How much of the suspension do you give?

For further assistance with calculations, please see Meriel Hutton's *Essential Calculation Skills for Nurses, Midwives and Healthcare Practitioners* (Open University Press 2009).

Multiple choice questions

Try answering these multiple choice questions to test what you have learned from reading this chapter. You can check your answers on page 199.

1 What is the mechanism of action of tetracycline antibiotics?

a) They inhibit folate use by the bacteria
b) They destroy the bacterial cell wall
c) They inhibit bacterial protein synthesis
d) They interfere with bacterial DNA

2 What is the drug of choice in treating tuberculosis?

a) Rifampacin
b) Gentamycin
c) Clindamycin
d) Chloramphenicol

3 Why should antacid medicines not be taken with certain antibiotics?

a) The body prefers to absorb antacids
b) Antacids slow down the movement of the bowel
c) They stop the antibiotic being absorbed by the body
d) They increase the side-effects of antibiotics

4 What is the mechanism of action of penicillins and cephalosporins?

a) They inhibit folate use by the bacteria
b) They constrict the bacterial cell wall
c) They inhibit bacterial protein synthesis
d) They interfere with bacterial DNA

5 Reverse transcriptase is associated with which virus?

a) Influenza
b) Herpes
c) Human cytomegalo
d) Human immunodeficiency

6 Aciclovir is used when treating

a) Poliomylitis
b) German measles
c) Influenza
d) Shingles

$\rightarrow$

←

7 Viruses are difficult to treat because

a) They reproduce in our cells
b) They have very thick walls
c) They are smaller than bacteria
d) The drugs are more expensive

8 Athlete's foot is an example of a

a) Mildew
b) True yeast
c) Mould
d) Yeast-like fungi

9 Which of the following drugs is most likely to lead to an infection with thrush?

a) Anticoagulant therapy
b) Morphine
c) Steroid medicines
d) Angiotensin converting enzyme inhibitors

10 Amphoteracin could be described as being

a) A newly-developed medicine
b) A synthetic antifungal agent
c) A harmless medicine
d) An antifungal antibiotic

Recommended further reading

AHRQ (Agency for Healthcare Research and Quality) (2000) Management of acute otitis media, report no. 15, http://archive.ahrq.gov.

Anonymous (2004) NT clinical: what you need to know about . . . antibiotics, *Nursing Times*, 100(19): 32.

Beckwith, S. and Franklin, P. (2007) *Oxford Handbook of Nurse Prescribing*. Oxford: Oxford University Press.

Brenner, G.M. and Stevens, C.W. (2009) *Pharmacology*, 3rd edn. Philadelphia, PA: Saunders Elsevier.

Campbell, S. (2004) Management of HIV/AIDS transmission in health care, *Nursing Standard*, 18(27): 33–5.

Clayton, B.D. (2009) *Basic Pharmacology for Nurses*, 15th edn. St Louis, MO: Mosby Elsevier.

Coben, D. and Atere-Roberts, E. (2005) *Calculations for Nursing and Healthcare*, 2nd edn. Basingstoke: Palgrave Macmillan.

DH (Department of Health) (2007) *Antibiotics: don't wear me out*. London: DH.

Downie, G., Mackenzie, J. and Williams, A. (2007) *Pharmacology and Medicines Management for Nurses*, 4th edn. Edinburgh: Churchill Livingstone.

Gatford, J.D. and Phillips, N. (2006) *Nursing Calculations*, 7th edn. Edinburgh: Churchill Livingstone Elsevier.

Karch, A.M. (2008) *Focus on Nursing Pharmacology*, 4th edn. Philadelphia, PA: Lippincott Williams & Wilkins.

Lapham, R. and Agar, H. (2009) *Drug Calculations for Nurses: A Step-by-step Approach*, 3rd edn. London: Arnold.

Mandel, B.K., Wilkins, E.G.L, Dunbar, E.M. and Mayon-White, R.T. (2004) *Lecture Notes on Infectious Diseases*, 6th edn. Malden, MA: Blackwell.

McKernan, C. (2008) Exploring the literature on delivering home IV therapy, *Nursing Times*, 104(34): 28–9.

NICE (National Institute for Health and Clinical Excellence) (2006) *Clinical Guideline 33: Tuberculosis.* London: NICE.

Pratt, R.J. (2003) *HIV & AIDS: A Foundation for Nursing and Healthcare Practice*, 5th edn. London: Arnold.

Simonson, T., Aarbakke, J., Kay, I., Coleman, I., Sinnott, P. and Lyssa, R. (2006) *Illustrated Pharmacology for Nurses.* London: Hodder Arnold.

WHO (World Health Organization) (2002) *Antimicrobial Resistance: A Report on Infectious Diseases*, www.who.int/infectious diseases report.

Zaidi, N., Tariq, M. and Breslin, D. (2009) Perioperative use of antibiotics in elective surgical patients: timing of administration, *Journal of Perioperative Practice*, 19(7): 225–7.

5

Anti-inflammatory drugs

Chapter contents

Learning objectives
Introduction
  Acute inflammation
  Chronic inflammation
Non-steroidal anti-inflammatory drugs
  Naproxen
Cyclo-oxygenase pathway 2 inhibitors
  Celecoxib
Aspirin
  Adverse effects
  Overdose
Paracetamol
Histamine
  Antihistamines

Steroids
  Administration
  Side-effects
Antirheumatoid drugs
  Sulfasalazine
  Gold compounds
  Penicillamine
  Methotrexate
  Chloroquine
  Leflunomide
Case studies
Key learning points
Calculations
Multiple choice questions
Recommended further reading

Learning objectives

After studying this chapter you should be able to:

- Describe acute and chronic inflammatory processes.
- Explain the mode of action of non-steroidal anti-inflammatory agents.
- Demonstrate an understanding of what is meant by cyclo-oxygenase pathway 2 inhibitors.
- Discuss the mode of action and adverse effects of aspirin.
- Define what is meant by the word 'histamine'.
- Describe the mode of action of antihistamine medication.
- Demonstrate an understanding of why steroid drugs are given, their routes of administration and side-effects.
- Explain what information the practitioner should give to a patient taking systemic steroid therapy.
- Define the condition rheumatoid arthritis.
- List three drugs that would be categorized as disease modifying antirheumatoid drugs.
- Correctly solve a number of drug calculations with regard to anti-inflammatory drugs.

Introduction

Inflammation is the body's response mechanism to cellular damage. Without the inflammatory response our bodies could not survive. Therefore, inflammation is a protective mechanism designed to rid the body of the cause of injury and prepare our tissues to rebuild themselves following injury.

The inflammatory response is a local reaction that involves release of antibacterial substances that defend the body from attack. The inflammatory process walls off the injured area so that toxins cannot affect the whole system. Finally, it puts in place the infrastructure that enables the body to heal itself and be restored to its normal functioning. In many ways, inflammation could be described as a *homeostatic mechanism*. The major signs and symptoms of inflammation are redness, pain, swelling, heat and loss of function. These are brought about by chemicals liberated by plasma proteins and cells. The plasma proteins and various white cells squeeze through the walls of capillary vessels and gain access to the site of tissue damage, infection or foreign body. This response is brought about by a variety of chemicals in the body which open up blood vessels (vasodilation) and act as messengers to summon white blood cells to the appropriate location. This messaging system is referred to as *chemotaxis*.

Inflammation can be classified as either acute or chronic. Both types will now be described.

Acute inflammation

An example of this would be an insect bite. The nature of acute inflammation is characterized by its rapid onset and short duration. This response is intended to remove debris from the tissue, such as micro-organisms and other particles of dead tissue. At the same time, the body sends messages to the bone marrow, which trigger a greater manufacture of phagocytic cells, particularly neutrophils, which have the ability to digest invading organisms. Finally, other chemical messengers summon these phagocytic cells from the area of damage by the process of chemotaxis.

One of the first chemicals to be released in the acute inflammatory response is called *histamine*.

This is released from a type of body cell called a *mast cell*. The role of histamine in the body is to produce vasodilation and increase the permeability of blood vessels. This in turn allows fluid and phagocytic cells to move from the intravascular fluid to the extravascular. The whole area of damage becomes flooded with fluid, plasma proteins and phagocytic cells. This fluid is called *acute inflammatory exudate* and its presence is detected by looking for the cardinal signs of inflammation discussed earlier.

The action of flooding the tissues with fluid and plasma proteins is important as it dilutes any toxins which may have been released, especially by bacteria. The excess fluid is drained away by a network of blind capillary-type vessels, which belong to the lymphatic system. This is important as small amounts of bacterial protein are exposed to lymphocytes which, in turn, produce antitoxins, which we call immunoglobulins. These are attracted to the area of cell injury to neutralize toxins further. A specific group of plasma proteins called the *complement group* assist the inflammatory response by attracting white cells by chemotaxis and promoting the amount of phagocytic cells made available to the body.

First into the battle zone are a group of granular leucocytes called *neutrophils*. These cells ingest small portions of dead tissue. They can do this as the cell contains packages of an enzyme that breaks down the bacterial walls. This is known as *lysozyme*. These packages release their contents and dissolve the debris. Neutrophil activity is limited, however, because they do not have the ability to make and store more of this enzyme. Therefore, once the neutrophil has used up all of its enzymes and phagocytosis is complete, the cell degenerates and dies.

Next into the arena of conflict come two types of agranular white blood cells – the *monocytes* and the *lymphocytes*. Once the monocyte enters the damaged area it undergoes a change in its structure, becoming a more specialist type of white cell known as a *macrophage*. These cells can mop up any cell debris or bacteria. Unlike neutrophils, they can replenish and package more lysozyme. Therefore, they can sustain the campaign against the

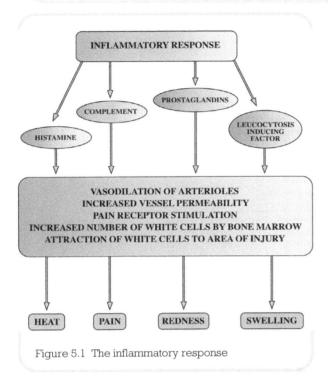

Figure 5.1 The inflammatory response

surrounding normal tissue. The inflammatory process itself will almost inevitably cause some damage to tissues by its efforts to save other tissues. This balancing act, therefore, has three possible end points:

- **Resolution.** Here there is complete healing and tissue repair.
- **Healing by repair.** Here the tissue is completely destroyed and now lacks the ability to regenerate. As a result, the tissue will be repaired by scar tissue. This tissue is fibrous in nature and lacks the specialization of the surrounding tissue.
- **Chronic inflammation.** This is brought about when the noxious material persists over an extended period of time, resulting in the continued destruction of tissue.

Chronic inflammation

As stated earlier, this usually arises when a noxious substance is not removed by the acute inflammatory process. There are times when chronic inflammation is not preceded by the acute inflammatory process. This is often the case in what are termed *autoimmune diseases*, where the body's defence mechanisms appear to be turned on themselves. Inflammation and destruction of normal body tissue by autoimmunoglobulins takes place. For some reason, the body is detecting some of its own tissue as foreign.

If the acute inflammatory phase cannot remove the foreign material, further tissue destruction takes place as the initial agent and the inflammatory response continue to battle it out. The body does make attempts to repair the damage, however, due to the continued battle between destruction and repair its efforts are hampered.

In chronic inflammation, the cells that are found at the site of injury differ from those for acute inflammation. The body is mounting a more specific defence and this is mirrored in the type of white cell found in the inflamed area. Rather than lots of neutrophils and macrophages being present, there are now large amounts of lymphocytes. Attempts to repair the tissues are now evident as fibrosis as

invading force. Their allies, the lymphocytes, are part of a more specific immune response and will have been alerted by removal of cellular materials via the lymphatic system. Specific cells will now have been created by the body to counteract these foreign proteins, which are called *antigens*. Two types of lymphocyte will have been created by the body: 'T' lymphocytes which naturally attack any foreign antigens, and 'B' lymphocytes which produce the immunoglobulins mentioned earlier which neutralize any toxins produced by the invading bacteria.

Once the area has been cleared, repair can take place. Cells that rebuild tissue, called *fibroblasts*, now start to proliferate and generate collagen, a protein necessary for wound repair. Also, a process known as *angiogenesis* can take place and blood vessels that have been destroyed in the damaged area start to grow again, supplying nutrients and oxygen to the newly forming tissues.

Acute inflammation can be seen as almost a balance between the amount of damage caused by the invading organisms and the damage caused by the body's response in terms of trying to safeguard

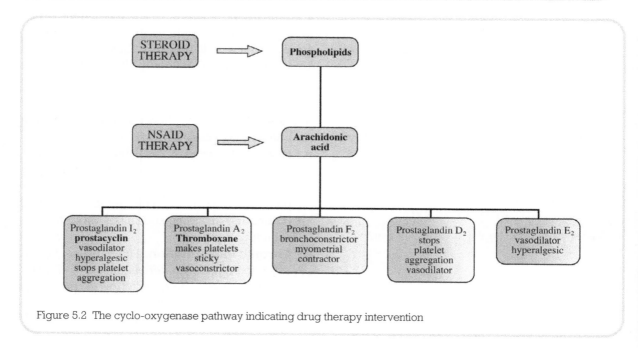

Figure 5.2 The cyclo-oxygenase pathway indicating drug therapy intervention

a result of thick bands of collagen fibres being laid down in a desperate attempt to heal the site of injury. In order for natural resolution to occur, the patient may need help via antibiotic therapy, having the foreign body removed or having nutritional support.

In order to understand the pharmacological action of certain anti-inflammatory drugs, we must probe deeper into physiology and focus our attention on a group of substances called *eicosanoids*. These include prostacyclin and thromboxane (which you will come across again in Chapter 6 on anticoagulants), and prostaglandins and leukotrienes. These agents are very important in triggering the inflammatory response and are formed when a fatty acid called *arachidonic acid* is liberated from a damaged cell membrane by action of an enzyme known as phospholipase.

The arachidonic acid acts by triggering two vitally important pathways, the cyclo-oxygenase pathway and lipoxygenase pathway. The cyclo-oxygenase pathway produces prostaglandins, whereas the lipoxygenase pathway leads to leukotriene formation. We will see in our exploration of anti-inflammatory drugs that some act on one pathway while others exert their effects on both.

Non-steroidal anti-inflammatory drugs

NSAIDs are a large and popular group of therapeutic agents. Their main use is as an analgesic to treat mild to moderate pain (see Chapter 3). Examples include ibuprofen, aspirin, naproxen and paracetamol. They are frequently prescribed for orthopaedic complaints, such as osteoarthritis and other musculoskeletal conditions. They are also a very popular OTC medication for minor aches and pains.

This group of drugs works by inhibiting the formation of prostaglandins. Prostaglandins are naturally occurring substances and are released when cell membranes are damaged in some way. They are responsible for dilation of vessels, causing redness and swelling. Some of them also sensitize the receptors that are responsible for us feeling the sensation of pain (see Chapter 3).

Let us now return to our discussion concerning the cyclo-oxygenase pathway. We have more than one cyclo-oxygenase system. Some researchers claim that there are as many as three. Cyclo-oxygenase pathways in most pharmacological texts are denoted by the prefix COX followed by the number of the pathway (e.g. COX1). The prostaglandins derived from COX1 are to do with the smooth running of body systems; in particular they help to maintain the protective mucous lining of the stomach and intestine. COX2 in comparison produces prostaglandins that facilitate pain and inflammation.

The vast number of current NSAIDs block both pathways. This is problematic as the drugs reduce the pain and inflammation associated with COX2 but also reduce the homeostatic function of COX1. This leads to a number of GI problems, the most significant of which is peptic ulceration. Often, oral administration of a prostaglandin substitute, such as misoprostol, may be used. This helps to ensure limited damage to the stomach mucosa. Also, some doctors will prescribe a drug known as a *proton pump inhibitor* which limits the amount of acid secretion by cells in the stomach wall. This in turn limits the risk of peptic ulcers forming. An example of a proton pump inhibitor would be omeprazole.

Another common side-effect of these drugs is the adverse reaction they can have on kidney function. Some prostaglandins in the COX1 pathway have an effect on the pressure of blood flow through the kidneys. As our kidneys need pressure in order to filter our blood, any drug that affects this fine balance can be potentially detrimental.

NSAIDs may also increase the risk of heart attacks, stroke and related conditions, which can be fatal. This risk may increase with duration of use and in patients who have underlying risk factors for heart and blood vessel conditions. NSAIDs should not be used for the treatment of pain resulting from coronary artery bypass graft surgery. They can cause an increased risk of serious, even fatal, stomach and intestinal adverse reactions such as bleeding, ulcers and perforation of the stomach or intestines. These events can occur at any time during treatment and without warning symptoms. Elderly patients are at greater risk for these types of reaction.

Clinical tip

Normal doses of NSAIDs in healthy individuals do not usually pose much of a risk. However, in patients that have other medical conditions such as heart failure, these drugs can cause acute kidney problems. Patients who are likely to react in an adverse way to this group of drugs should have their blood checked at regular intervals for signs of renal insufficiency.

In the introduction to this chapter we described the chemicals that cause inflammation. NSAIDs reduce this inflammatory response by dampening down processes such as vasodilation, the formation of oedema as vessels become more permeable and, finally, pain. It is thought that this class of drug interferes with COX2 but has the disadvantage of interfering with COX1.

Naproxen

This is a commonly used NSAID in the reduction of pain, fever, inflammation and stiffness associated with conditions such as arthritis and ankylosing spondylitis (a chronic arthritis of the spine). Naproxen is often one of the first choices when treating an inflammatory condition because it is very effective with relatively few side-effects. However, ibuprofen is still the safest (see Chapter 3).

The dose of naproxen will vary depending on the condition it is being used to treat. However the usual adult dose is 250–500mg twice daily. Because of potential effects on the gastric lining a drug such as misoprostol may also be used.

Naproxen is associated with several suspected or probable interactions that affect the action of other drugs. For example, it may increase the blood levels of lithium by reducing the excretion of lithium by the kidneys. Increased levels of lithium may lead to lithium toxicity. Naproxen may reduce the blood pressure-lowering effects of blood pressure medication because prostaglandins play a role in the regulation of blood pressure.

When naproxen is used in combination with methotrexate or aminoglycosides (e.g. gentamicin) the blood levels of the methotrexate or amino-glycoside may increase, presumably because the elimination from the body is reduced. This can lead to more methotrexate or aminoglycoside-related side-effects. Individuals taking oral blood thinners or anticoagulants, for example, warfarin, should avoid naproxen because it also thins the blood, and excessive blood thinning may lead to bleeding.

There are no adequate studies of naproxen in pregnant women. Therefore, it is not recommended during pregnancy, even though the concentration of naproxen in breast milk is very low and therefore breastfeeding while taking this drug is probably not harmful to the infant.

Cyclo-oxygenase pathway 2 inhibitors

It would appear from our description of COX1 as good prostaglandin formation and COX2 as bad prostaglandin formation that an obvious solution to the problem would be to come up with a group of drugs that first inhibited the COX2 pathway. Indeed, this is what has happened. This search for COX2 specific drugs resulted in a number of early forerunners – valdecoxib, celecoxib and rofecoxib. However, in 2004 rofecoxib (VIOXX) was withdrawn voluntarily from the market due to studies which suggested that it increased the risk of myocardial infarction and stroke. These side-effects are linked to prostaglandin inhibition.

Certain prostaglandins are important for the balance in our bodies that allows our blood to clot (see Chapter 6). This fine balance is upset in a number of people, leading to increased risk of thrombosis. Hence, valdecoxib was also withdrawn voluntarily from the market in April 2005 because of concerns that it was causing more frequent serious skin reactions than other drugs in the same class. Drugs of this type are still under review, however it is hoped that refinement of this class of medication will lead to new formulations being made available in the future.

Celecoxib

Celecoxib belongs to a new generation of NSAIDs that selectively block the action of COX2. This means that it stops the production of inflammatory prostaglandins without stopping the production of prostaglandins that protect the stomach and intestines. It therefore reduces pain and inflammation, but is less likely than traditional NSAIDs to cause side-effects on the stomach and intestines (although such side-effects are still possible).

This medicine is commonly used for various types of joint and muscular conditions, such as arthritis. The lowest effective dose should be used for each patient. For the management of osteoarthritis, the dose is usually 100mg twice daily or 200mg as a single dose. For rheumatoid arthritis, the dose is usually 100 or 200mg twice daily.

Celecoxib, like other NSAIDs may cause serious stomach and intestinal ulcers that can occur at any time during treatment. It does not interfere with the function of the blood platelets and, as a result, does not reduce clotting and lead to increased bleeding time like other NSAIDs. Allergic reactions can occur with celecoxib. Individuals who have developed allergic reactions (e.g. rash, itching, difficulty breathing) from sulfonamides, aspirin or other NSAIDs may experience an allergic reaction to celecoxib and should not take this drug.

Fluconazole (diflucan) increases the concentration of celecoxib in the body by preventing the elimination of celecoxib in the liver. Therefore, treatment with celecoxib should be initiated at the lowest recommended doses in patients who are taking fluconazole. As diflucan can be obtained from a pharmacist, it is important always to ask the patient about other medicines they may be taking prior to dispensing.

Aspirin

Aspirin is a very versatile drug (see also Chapters 3 and 6). In terms of its anti-inflammatory properties, it is used in the treatment of rheumatic fever, rheumatoid arthritis and other inflammatory joint conditions. Aspirin is another drug which blocks the COX1 pathway, but also inhibits the COX2 pathway. Furthermore, aspirin has been found to have effects on the release of energy at a cellular level, especially in the liver and cartilaginous tissue. It induces chemicals that enable white cells to fight infections more effectively.

Aspirin is a weak acid drug that will readily be absorbed in the stomach due to its acid environment. However, much of the absorption takes place in the ileum, the third part of the small intestine, due to its large surface area.

Aspirin is taken orally and can be obtained in a soluble form, where it is mixed with calcium carbonate and citric acid. This aids its rate of absorption into the body.

Adverse effects

Some of the adverse effects caused by aspirin are similar to those previously described as side-effects of NSAIDs – for example, GI complaints. In addition to these are a group of symptoms caused by central nervous system disruption. These include dizziness, tinnitus, loss of hearing, visual disturbances and headache. The drug should not be given to children as it can cause a life-threatening disorder called Reyes syndrome.

Overdose

Overdose with aspirin has serious consequences. More serious symptoms of poisoning include high body temperature (hyperthermia), increased respiratory rate (tachypnoea), metabolic acidosis, confusion, cerebral oedema and coma. Aspirin overdose is still classified as a medical emergency.

Paracetamol

This drug has only a relatively weak anti-inflammatory effect due to action on a reported third COX pathway. Its use is described more fully in Chapter 3.

Histamine

Histamine is a chemical liberated by the body, which contributes to the inflammatory response and is found in most body tissue. However, the lungs, skin and GI tract have high concentrations. It is also found in cells, namely mast cells and basophils. Histamine also occurs in cells in the stomach and certain neurons in the brain.

Histamine has an action on a number of different receptors. As we will be discussing drugs that affect histamine receptors, it is necessary to describe how histamine acts on the bodily systems that contain these receptors. Smooth muscle, except that in the cardiovascular system, contracts; the blood vessels have the opposite action of dilating. H-receptors also bring about an increase in the permeability of blood capillaries.

Antihistamines

The term 'antihistamine' usually refers to drugs that block the action of histamine on H-receptors. This class of drug affects various inflammatory and allergic responses. If we block the body's ability to respond to the release of histamine then the inflammatory response, in terms of vasodilation and increased permeability of vessels, will no longer take place or will be modified.

Most drugs in this category are given orally as they are well absorbed by the body. Generally, most reach a peak in the plasma after one or two hours. These drugs are well distributed throughout the body and some do not cross the BBB and, therefore, cause less sedation than those that do.

Cyclizine, dimenhydrinate and cinnarizine do cross the BBB and can be used for motion sickness. Non-sedating antihistamines, such as terfenadine, are mainly used for hay fever and mild allergic reactions. The drug can, however, rarely cause serious cardiac problems. Some non-sedating drugs in this category can now be purchased as OTC medicines, for example loratadine and cetirizine. Some sedating drugs in this group can can actually be used for this effect, for example, promethazine. However, using the central nervous system actions of antihistamines can be problematic. They may well cause sedation and stop motion sickness, but they will also produce other central nervous system side-effects that are less useful, for example, dizziness, tinnitus and tiredness. The most significant side-effects of antihistamines at a peripheral, rather than a central level, are dryness of the mouth, blurred vision and, more rarely, constipation and retention of urine.

Steroids

Steroid hormones include a group known as *glucocorticoids*. These are secreted by an area of the adrenal cortex known as the *zona fasciculate*. Glucocorticoids are involved in the body's response to stress. First, they have a pronounced effect on carbohydrate and protein use. The hormones cause a decrease in the uptake of glucose by the body's cells and an increase in glucose production via the breakdown of proteins (gluconeogenesis). This leads to a net increase in the blood sugar (hyperglycaemia). At the same time, the body stores more glucose as glycogen in the liver. Protein use is affected as there is a decrease in the production of protein by the cells but an increase in protein breakdown, which is particularly evident in muscle tissue. Use of fats is also affected by glucocorticoids as they permit fatty tissue to be laid down in a certain way.

Glucocorticoids also affect certain electrolytes within the body. Sodium is retained at the expense of potassium, which is lost via the kidneys. Calcium is another example of a body chemical affected by glucocorticoid activity, as glucocorticoids tend to lower the rate of absorption by the GI tract and increase its loss via the kidneys.

If levels of glucocorticoid remain high in the plasma, this has a negative feedback effect on the hypothalamus and pituitary gland. Basically, the body ceases to stimulate the adrenal cortex to produce these substances, and over a period of time this will lead to a shrinking of the adrenal cortical area.

The important role of glucocorticoids as far as this chapter is concerned is their powerful anti-inflammatory and immunosuppressive effects. They not only stop initial redness, pain, heat and swelling but also affect the healing and repair process. They have the ability to stop all types of inflammatory response whether caused by physical stimuli or inappropriate immune responses in the body.

Glucocorticoids have a direct action on the cells involved in the inflammatory response, for example, neutrophils, macrophages and fibroblasts. They also have a direct action on the chemicals responsible for inflammation itself (e.g. COX2 and histamine). If you are wondering why the body would produce such hormones in response to what is a natural part of the healing process, it is thought that the production of glucocorticoids is a homeostatic mechanism aimed at keeping in check the powerful defence systems of the body.

Whatever the reason for their production, glucocorticoids can be harnessed to help treat conditions where hypersensitivity or unwanted inflammatory processes present. This group of drugs can therefore be used in a range of conditions from autoimmune disease and organ rejection following transplantation to hay fever and skin conditions. However, their ability to suppress the normal inflammatory response has consequences in the masking of infections and a decrease the potential healing properties of all tissue.

Administration

Glucocorticoids can be given a number of ways. Most types can be administered by mouth and all can be given via the IM or IV routes. They can be applied in a cream to the skin or given as eye drops or nasal sprays. They may be administered directly into joint spaces (intra-articularly) or into the lungs by means of an aerosol. Examples of glucocorticoid drugs are prednisilone, hydrocortisone, dexamethasone and beclomethasone.

Side-effects

Side-effects are a very important issue, however, these are more likely when these drugs are given systemically rather than locally or when they are prescribed in high doses over an extended period of time. Side-effects are not normally seen when these drugs are given as replacement therapy. Patients on long continued treatment with glucocorticoids are obviously at risk of developing serious side-effects. As the body's blood sugar is constantly elevated, the body develops a secondary diabetic condition. Also, as sodium is retained by the body, so is water, therefore increasing blood volume and leading to a hypertensive state.

Glucocorticoid actions of lowering the calcium plasma level lead to the body homeostatically replacing this from the bones. This in turn leads to osteoporosis and potential occurrence of fractures.

Glucose being formed by proteins leads to muscular weakness and, in children, can affect growth.

However, this is unlikely unless the treatment is extended to six months or more.

As the person's ability to fight infection is compromised, infection can go undetected. Any infection must be treated early with antibiotics and an increased dose of steroid to compensate for the body's natural response. A particularly problematic side-effect is the inability of wounds to heal. This can lead to extensive long-term therapies being instigated to treat traumatic injuries.

Box 5.1 Common side-effects of steroids

Secondary hypertension
Euphoria
Hirsutism
Moon-shaped face
Masked infection
Osteoporosis
Adrenal atrophy
Peptic ulceration
Thinning of the skin
Generalized weakness
Secondary diabetes
Obesity
Striae
Oedema
Poor wound healing

Clinical tip

Normal doses of steroids in healthy individuals do not usually pose much of a risk. However, in patients that may have other medical conditions, for example, heart failure, these drugs can cause acute kidney problems. Patients who are likely to react in an adverse way to this group of drugs should have their blood checked at regular intervals for signs of renal insufficiency.

The patient must also be educated regarding the risks of suddenly stopping their medication. If the body has stopped stimulating the adrenal cortex, it will lose its ability to make its own corticosteroids. Therefore, any sudden withdrawal will lead to a gross insufficiency and the patient may well enter what is called a 'steroidal crisis'. Patients should be phased off their medication slowly to allow the body to recover its natural abilities. This normally takes about two months, although it may take much longer.

All patients receiving long-term therapy are advised to carry a card stating that they are undergoing steroid treatment, which must not be stopped abruptly. They should also inform their dentist about their treatment.

Antirheumatoid drugs

Arthritis is inflammation of the joints. Rheumatoid arthritis is a fairly common condition and affects about affects around 400,000 people in the UK. Unlike osteoarthritis, which tends to occur as we get older, rheumatoid arthritis can develop at any age, but usually starts in middle adult life, between the ages of 40 and 60. It affects women more than men with a 3:1 ratio.

Rheumatoid arthritis is thought to be an autoimmune disease. In people with this condition, antibodies are formed against the synovial membrane (the capsule which surrounds each joint). This causes inflammation in and around the affected joints. Over time, the inflammation causes damage to the joint, the cartilage and parts of the bone involved in forming the joint.

We have already discussed two classes of drugs that are used in this condition, namely NSAIDs and glucocorticoids. However, the group of drugs most frequently used in treating this disease goes under the umbrella term of 'disease-modifying antirheumatoid drugs' (DMARDs).

The DMARD group includes a variety of drugs with differing chemical structures and, therefore, modes of action, such as sulfasalazine, gold compounds, penicillamine, chloroquine, methotrexate and leflunomide. The antirheumatoid actions of the drugs in this category were discovered mostly by accident: we know that they work but have no conclusive evidence to suggest why. DMARDs improve patients' lives by reducing the swelling and tenderness in the joints, and while some years ago this class of drugs was usually used as a last resort it is now usual to start a DMARD as soon as possible after diagnosis has been made, in order to limit the disease as much as possible.

Clinical tip

Sometimes DMARDs have no immediate effect on symptoms and it may take up to six months before the patient starts to feel the benefit. Therefore, it is important to educate the patient regarding continuing to take the drugs as prescribed even if no effect is felt at first.

Sulfasalazine

Sulfasalazine is a pro-drug, which means that it is not active in the form in which it is given. The drug is broken down into two active components by bacteria that live in the bowel: 5 aminosalicylic acid and sulfapyridine. It is not clear which of these agents is responsible for the beneficial immunosuppressant effect.

GI side-effects are common and include nausea, vomiting and loss of appetite (anorexia). Dizziness can also be a troubling side-effect for a number of patients. More serious side-effects include a drop in white cells in the body (leucopenia). Skin rashes and reactions to sunlight (photosensitivity) can also occur. As with any drug, sulfasalazine should be used with caution in patients who have kidney disease, when the dose may need to be reduced.

Gold compounds

The earliest use of gold for medicinal purposes can be traced back to Chinese medicine in 2500

BC. As with sulfasalazine, the effect of gold compounds occurs slowly. The patient may not feel any benefit from the medication for a period of three or four months. However, after this time patients' pain and joint swelling starts to lessen. This is mirrored by a slowing down of the bone and cartilage damage within the joint. The mode of action of gold compounds is not certain at the present time.

Gold is usually given as either sodium aurothiomalate or auranofin. Sodium aurothiomalate is administered by deep IM injection whereas auranofin is given orally. Auranofin also has other advantages in that the levels of gold in the plasma are less but are maintained for longer; therefore, less gold accumulates in the tissues of the body. This means that the kidneys have to excrete less gold and, therefore, do not run the risk of being damaged by high concentrations of this metal. However, the drawback of using auranofin ('oral gold') is that it is not as effective in symptom control compared with aurothiomalate. Aurothiomalate has the ability to control symptoms better than its oral counterpart but comes at a price to the patient's biological systems, in particular the risk of kidney destruction (nephrotoxicity).

Clinical tip

Some patients may develop a number of serious adverse effects to gold compounds that may mean the therapy must be stopped. These are: severe mouth ulcers (stomatitis), kidney damage, blood disorders and major brain and liver disorders. The patient, nurse and doctor need to be vigilant for adverse signs and symptoms as early cessation means that these serious side-effects can be avoided.

Penicillamine

This drug was discovered in the 1950s as being in the urine of patients who had taken penicillin. The drug itself has no antibiotic properties and is used to treat rheumatoid arthritis due to its immunosuppressive effects. The exact nature of its action is still being debated. However, it is thought to reduce the number of circulating T-lymphocytes and macrophages. It also affects chemotactic agents and prevents an important protein called collagen from maturing. Like most of the DMARDs it takes weeks or months before the patient feels any benefit from the drug.

Penicillamine is given orally, beginning on a low dose which is increased every two months. The maximum dose is about 1500mg per day. The reason for this gradual dosing regime is to avoid unwanted side-effects because at high doses as many as one in four patients has to stop taking the medication due to unwanted effects.

As with many of the drugs in this section, side-effects include anorexia, nausea and vomiting. Some patients develop a loss of taste because the drug binds to zinc, which is important in this sensation. Rashes and stomatitis are common and serious side-effects include blood disorders such as leucopenia, anaemia and thrombocytopenia.

As penicillamine binds to certain metals (chelation) it should not be given to patients who are taking iron supplements, gold and antacids that contain aluminium or magnesium. Taking this drug also makes the body demand more vitamin B$_6$ (pyridoxine). Therefore, you may find the doctor or nurse practitioner prescribing a supplement.

Methotrexate

Methotrexate works on DNA, the genetic material within the nucleus of a cell. As with most drugs in this classification, it is not known how exactly methotrexate works in relation to rheumatoid arthritis, but empirically it has been shown to reduce the amount of inflammation and slow the progression of the disease. It is usually the drug of choice as a first-line treatment following diagnosis. The drug has fewer side-effects than others in this group and because of its favourable results patients are more likely to be concordant (continue to take the medication).

Studies have suggested that when methotrexate is given alongside another DMARD, disease and, therefore, symptom progression is much less marked than when giving one drug only. Combi-

nation therapy may also allow for lower doses of individual drugs to be given.

Side-effects include nausea, stomatitis, diarrhoea, fatigue and mild inflammation of the liver. As the drug affects the body's ability to fight infection, the patient should be educated to report signs and symptoms, such as sore throat, shortness of breath and frequency of mictiration to a health professional. Low blood cell counts are less likely with this drug than others in this group. Rare side-effects such as liver damage and lung damage may occur.

Chloroquine

This drug is used mainly in the treatment of malaria. However, it is shown to reduce progression of disease in rheumatoid arthritis. The drug is generally used in milder cases of the disease or in combination with other DMARDs. It takes about three to six months to show any reported effects and minor side-effects are similar to those reported in other DMARDs, such as nausea, diarrhoea and rashes.

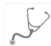

Clinical tip

More serious side-effects from chloroquine are ophthalmologic in nature. Prolonged use may lead patients to complain of problems with their peripheral and night-time vision. If patients are prescribed the drug, they should be advised to have a baseline eye test and repeat this on a six-monthly to yearly basis.

Leflunomide

This drug is thought to work on the cell's DNA and RNA. The immune cells cannot function or reproduce effectively due to the drug's effect. Hence, leflunomide reduces inflammation in the joints, as well as slowing down progressive bone erosion and joint deformity.

The drug can be taken orally and comes in preparations of 10, 20 and 100mg tablets. The usual dose is 100mg daily for the first three days, then 20mg daily, or 10mg if side-effects appear. These include nausea, diarrhoea and rashes. More severe side-effects are hypertension, chest pain and abnormal heartbeats. Like many of the immunosuppressant DMARDs, leflunomide can mask infections. Liver damage is also a possibility and if liver enzyme tests remain abnormal the drug should be discontinued.

This drug has not been studied adequately as part of combination therapy for someone with rheumatoid arthritis. Therefore, at the present time prescribing with other DMARDs is contraindicated.

Case studies

① Radu Beligan, a 28-year-old professional musician, has been admitted to the ward for medical treatment following an exacerbation of his ulcerative colitis. On admission he was pale with obvious signs of weight loss. During his stay on the ward it is decided to commence oral steroid medication. You have been asked by your mentor to help prepare the patient for discharge. What information would you give to Radu with regard to his new medication with reference to:

- The action of steroids on the body?
- The side-effects?
- Any other information?

② Louise Mason is 12 years old. She has juvenile chronic arthritis which has been treated with ibuprofen. The doctor now wishes to give her a 'short burst' of high dose steroid to bridge her transition onto methotrexate. You have to explain to Louise and her concerned parents how these drugs work and why the steroids need to be given as a bridge from one set of medication to another. How would you put the following information into terms that Louise and her parents will understand:

- The mode of action of these three classes of medicine?
- The need for Louise to maintain drug therapy between stopping one drug and starting another?
- The possible side-effects that the high dose steroid treatment will have?

Key learning points

Introduction

➤ Inflammation is a protective mechanism.
➤ The inflammatory response is a local reaction.
➤ The cardinal signs and symptoms of inflammation are redness, pain, swelling, heat and loss of function.
➤ Acute inflammation is characterized by rapid onset and short duration.
➤ Histamine is released and is a vasodilator.
➤ Area of damage becomes flooded with exudate.

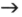

- ➢ Complement proteins are involved in chemotaxis.
- ➢ A variety of leucocytes are attracted to the area.
- ➢ Eventually repair takes place.
- ➢ Chronic inflammation occurs when noxious substances are not removed by the acute phase.
- ➢ Large amounts of lymphocytes are found in the area of chronic inflammation.
- ➢ Attempts to repair tissue often result in fibrosis.
- ➢ Inflammation is caused by the liberation of arachidonic acid.
- ➢ Cyclo-oxygenase and lipo-oxygenase pathways are triggered.

Non-steroidal anti-inflammatory drugs

- ➢ Popular group of drugs.
- ➢ Work by inhibiting prostaglandin formation.
- ➢ Stop the initiation of the cyclo-oxygenase pathway.
- ➢ Cause renal and gastrointestinal side-effects.

Naproxen

- ➢ Is often one of the first choices when treating an inflammatory condition.
- ➢ May increase the blood levels of lithium.
- ➢ May increase the levels of methotrexate or aminoglycoside.
- ➢ Is associated with the smallest overall cardiovascular risks but may increase the risk of heart attacks, stroke and related conditions.

Cyclo-oxygenase pathway 2 inhibitors

- ➢ New set of drugs.
- ➢ Some problems initially resulting in withdrawal of some drugs from the market.
- ➢ Sometimes have serious side-effects due to prostaglandin inhibition.

Celecoxib

- ➢ Commonly used for joint and muscular conditions, such as arthritis.
- ➢ Like other NSAIDs may cause serious stomach and intestinal ulcers.

Aspirin

- ➢ Versatile drug.
- ➢ Blocks COX1.
- ➢ Is a weak acid which is well absorbed in the stomach.
- ➢ Should not be given to children.
- ➢ Causes many side-effects.
- ➢ Serious in overdose.

Histamine

➤ Found in high concentrations in the lungs, skin and GI tract.
➤ Released by mast cells.
➤ Brings about vasodilation and increased permeability.

Antihistamines

➤ Block action of histamine.
➤ Modify inflammatory response.
➤ Some are used to treat motion sickness, some for allergic responses.
➤ Some have more sedating effects than others.
➤ Side-effects include dryness of mouth, blurred vision, constipation and retention of urine.

Steroids

➤ Produced naturally by the adrenal cortex.
➤ Involved in the body's response to stress.
➤ Effect metabolism of fats, carbohydrates and proteins.
➤ Steroid hormones also affect certain electrolytes (e.g. calcium and sodium).
➤ Giving replacement steroids causes atrophy of the adrenal gland.
➤ Steroids are powerful anti-inflammatory agents.
➤ Have a direct action on all cells involved in the inflammatory response.
➤ Have many side-effects.
➤ May be given by a number of routes.
➤ Can cause secondary diabetes and hypertension.
➤ Can cause osteoporosis and fractures.
➤ Can cause infection to go undetected and wounds not to heal.
➤ Patients must carry a card and have good discharge advice.

Antirheumatoid drugs

➤ Rheumatoid arthritis is an autoimmune condition.
➤ Drugs used in its treatment are called disease-modifying anti-rheumatoid drugs (DMARDs).
➤ These drugs improve patients' lives by reducing swelling and tenderness in the joints.
➤ Examples are methotrexate, penicillamine and gold.
➤ Often patients have no improvement for many months.
➤ Side-effects are serious and mainly lead to the patient discontinuing treatment.

Calculations

1   A doctor has prescribed 30mg of prednisolone. You have 5mg tablets on the ward. How many should you give?

2   5mg of prednisolone is equivalent to 20mg of hydrocortisone. How many 5mg prednisolone tablets is equivalent to a dose of 100mg of hydrocortisone?

3   A 3-year-old who weighs 13.5kg has been prescribed ibuprofen 5mg per kg three times daily. Ibuprofen is available as a suspension of 100mg in 5ml. How much should the child receive on each occasion?

4   The doctor prescribes a patient nefopam 60mg by intramuscular injection. This drug is available as 20mg in 1ml. How many ml do you give the patient?

5   A patient requires 85mg of cortisone. The stock ampoule is 100mg in 5ml. How much volume is required?

6   The doctor prescribes a patient 1g of paracetamol. The tablets come in 500mg. How many tablets will you give?

7   A child weighing 30kg is prescribed 80mg per kg per day of paracetamol to be given every six hours. What is the size of each dose?

8   Methylprednisolone 60mg is to be given by IM injection. Available is a solution of 80mg in 1ml. How much do you draw up?

9   The qualified nurse on the ward has to prepare hydrocortisone 400mg for IV injection. She has ampoules consisting of a solution 250mg in 2ml. How many ml will she draw up for you to check?

10   Phenergan 25mg IM is prescribed for a patient. The stock on the ward is 50mg in 1ml. How much fluid do you draw into the syringe?

For further assistance with calculations, please see Meriel Hutton's *Essential Calculation Skills for Nurses, Midwives and Healthcare Practitioners* (Open University Press 2009).

Multiple choice questions

Try answering these multiple choice questions to test what you have learned from reading this chapter. You can check your answers on page 200.

1 The role of histamine in the inflammatory response is

a) To attract white blood cells to the area of inflammation
b) To increase the amount of neutrophils being produced
c) To produce immunoglobulins
d) To produce vasodilation and increase permeability of blood vessels

←

2 In chronic inflammation what type of cells are found at the site of injury?

a) Lymphocytes
b) Neutrophils
c) Macrophages
d) Erythrocytes

3 Why do NSAIDs affect kidney function?

a) Because they are excreted by the kidneys
b) Because they cause widespread vasodilation
c) Because they interfere with normal homeostatic functions of prostaglandins
d) Because they are toxic to the kidney tubules

4 Why would you not give aspirin to children?

a) Because it could cause problems with the liver and brain
b) Because it is not effective in children
c) Because it damages the child's kidneys
d) Because the drug has been superseded by modern drugs

5 Steroid hormones are produced by

a) The hypothalamus
b) The adrenal glands
c) The thymus gland
d) The spleen

6 Steroids may cause secondary hypertension because

a) They lower calcium levels
b) They cause glycogen to break down to glucose
c) They retain sodium
d) They retain potassium

7 Why should steroid drugs not suddenly be discontinued?

a) Because only a consultant physician can do this
b) Because this should only be carried out in hospital
c) The body becomes tolerant to the drug
d) The body needs time to recover its natural steroid-making capacity

8 Which of the following is a DMARD?

a) Prostacyclin
b) Penicillin
c) Penicillamine
d) Paracetamol

→

9 What is the drug of choice in treating rheumatoid arthritis?

a) Gold compounds
b) Methotrexate
c) Sulfasalazine
d) Chloroquine

10 What is the mode of action of DMARDs?

a) Mostly it is unknown
b) They promote secretion of steroid hormones
c) They inhibit stem cell production
d) They inhibit action of white cells

Recommended further reading

Beckwith, S. and Franklin, P. (2007) *Oxford Handbook of Nurse Prescribing*. Oxford: Oxford University Press.

Brenner, G.M. and Stevens, C.W. (2006) *Pharmacology*, 2nd edn. Philadelphia, PA: Saunders Elsevier.

Clayton, B.D. (2009) *Basic Pharmacology for Nurses*, 15th edn. St Louis, MO: Mosby Elsevier.

Coben, D. and Atere-Roberts, E. (2005) *Calculations for Nursing and Healthcare*, 2nd edn. Basingstoke: Palgrave Macmillan.

Downie, G., Mackenzie, J. and Williams, A. (2007) *Pharmacology and Medicines Management for Nurses*, 4th edn. Edinburgh: Churchill Livingstone.

Gatford, J.D. and Phillips, N. (2006) *Nursing Calculations*, 7th edn. Edinburgh: Churchill Livingstone Elsevier.

Jordan, S. (2001) Non-steroidal anti-inflammatory drugs: clinical issues, *Nursing Standard*, 15(23).

Jordan, S. (2004) Prescription drugs, uses and effects: non-steroidal anti-inflammatory drugs, *Nursing Standard*, 18(23).

Karch, A.M. (2008) *Focus on Nursing Pharmacology*, 4th edn. Philadelphia, PA: Lippincott Williams & Wilkins.

Lapham, R. and Agar, H. (2003) *Drug Calculations for Nurses: A Step-by-step Approach*, 2nd edn. London: Arnold.

Middleton, C. (2003) Non-steroidal anti-inflammatory drugs: indications for use, *Nursing Times*, 99(16): 30–2.

Simonson, T., Aarbakke, J., Kay, I., Coleman, I., Sinnott, P. and Lyssa, R. (2006) *Illustrated Pharmacology for Nurses*. London: Hodder Arnold.

Trounce, J. (2000) *Clinical Pharmacology for Nurses*, 16th edn. New York: Churchill Livingstone.

Anticoagulant therapy

6

Chapter contents

Learning objectives
Introduction
  Constriction of the blood vessel
  Formation of a platelet plug
  Formation of the fibrin/blood clot
  Dissolving of the fibrin clot
**Blood clotting and the development
  of thrombosis**
Drugs that act on the clotting cascade
  Vitamin K
  Heparin
  Low molecular weight heparins
  Enoxaparin
  Hirudin

Warfarin
Future anticoagulant therapy
Antiplatelet drugs
  Aspirin
  Clopidogrel
  Abciximab
Fibrinolytic drugs
  Streptokinase
  Alteplase
Case study
Key learning points
Calculations
Multiple choice questions
Recommended further reading

Learning objectives

After studying this chapter you should be able to:

- Describe the four processes involved in normal blood clotting.
- List the factors that increase the likelihood of thrombosis occurring.
- Identify at least six drugs that act on the clotting cascade.
- Compare the mode of action of aspirin, heparin and warfarin.
- List the drugs that would be used to reverse the effects of heparin and warfarin.
- Define what is meant by the term 'international normalized ratio'.
- Describe the information given to a patient who is taking anticoagulant therapy, in particular warfarin.
- Demonstrate an understanding of fibrinolytic drugs and suggest in which circumstances they may be given.
- Identify a circumstance when a fibrinolytic drug would be contraindicated.
- Correctly solve a number of drug calculations with regard to anticoagulant therapy.

Introduction

Blood clotting is a normal homeostatic mechanism, the purpose of which is to prevent the loss of blood from the cardiovascular system and to ensure that blood vessels remain intact. This mechanism works very well in preventing haemorrhage from smaller blood vessels (e.g. capillaries, arterioles and venules). However, the mechanism is overwhelmed if bleeding occurs from the large vessels such as major veins or arteries. If such bleeding occurs, interventions from a first aid, medical or surgical perspective have to be employed in order to control the bleeding.

The word used for stopping haemorrhage from the body is *haemostasis* and, as stated above, is a normal homeostatic function of the body. The blood and damaged blood vessels have the ability to release components which work together to form a plug of solid matter which blocks the tear in the blood vessel. Haemostasis is divided into four processes, which will now be outlined.

Constriction of the blood vessel

Following the tearing of a blood vessel, the body reflexively constricts the size of the vessel, which also leads to the contraction of the severed ends. The constriction of vessels spreads to affect other local small vessels. The blood flow through these small vessels is now reduced and this allows the platelets and the plasma to come into contact with the damaged area of the blood vessel. When this occurs the body is setting in motion a state of events, the first being a reduction in the likelihood of the plug of platelets being washed away.

Formation of a platelet plug

Damage to the wall of a blood vessel exposes proteins within the vessel wall. These are collagen and elastin fibres and lie underneath the thin inside layer of the vessel. The exposure of these important proteins causes platelets to adhere to the site of the injury. Adhesion of the platelets to themselves and the site of the injury is further helped by one of the *plasma clotting factors* called factor VIII.

The process of platelet adhesion is reversible up to a point. Once the platelets have released the granules which they contain, white blood cells begin to stick to the platelets. During this build up of the foundation of the clot, the platelets also release a substance known as thromboxane (TXA_2). This has two effects: first, it increases the ability of the cells to stick together; second, it makes the blood vessel smaller by vasoconstriction. At this point it should be noted that the cells that have been exposed under the intima lining of the blood vessels start to produce a substance known as prostacyclin. This works in the opposite way to thromboxane in that it stimulates vasodilation and stops the process of the cells sticking together. This is an important point as certain drugs are given to affect the balance between thromboxane and prostacyclin (e.g. Dipyridamole).

As the platelet cells continue to stick together, they release a platelet factor which acts as a platform on which various blood clotting factors can bind. The foundation is now secured for the next process to begin.

Formation of the fibrin/blood clot

The essential end point of this process is an insoluble protein called *fibrin* which will plug the tear in the vessel wall. Insoluble fibrin lays down a mesh of white fibres which stick to each other and to tissue cells. This mesh traps other blood cells and more platelets. The clot gradually constricts, squeezing out any serum and leaving a solid but elastic plug.

To get to this end point, the blood and platelets have to go through a complex chain reaction. Each phase of this reaction is brought about by what are called 'plasma clotting factors' (always referred to using Roman numerals: see Table 6.1).

This cascade of events can be triggered in two distinct ways. First, damaged cells release a substance called *thromboplastin* or factor III. As thromboplastin is not part of the blood, this blood clotting pathway is known as the *extrinsic pathway*. The extrinsic pathway is therefore triggered by events such as physical injury to the blood vessels. The second triggering mechanism comes from contact of the blood with exposed collagen fibres, which are not usually exposed as they lie under the inner surface of the blood vessel. However, if damage occurs to this delicate lining, collagen fibres come into contact with blood products and the clotting mechanism commences. This particular set of events is known as the *intrinsic pathway*. The triggering of the extrinsic pathway would come from pathological states such as atherosclerosis (fatty deposits being laid down in the walls of arteries).

The key step in both systems is activation of a plasma factor called factor X. These systems work together to ensure that the body produces large enough amounts of thrombin to be effective in stemming blood loss.

A point to remember here is that the blood is thought to contain natural inhibitors of the clotting factors. It is these inhibitors that are believed to stop widespread clotting from taking place, therefore localizing events. The best known of these natural anticoagulants is *antithrombin III*.

Dissolving of the fibrin clot

Dissolving of a clot takes place much more slowly than does the building of one and the slow removal of the clot is part of life's normal process. Fibrin is dissolved by a substance known as *plasmin*. This product is not normally present in the plasma but is derived from an inactive protein called *plasminogen*. Plasminogen can be activated by a number of triggers, for example, plasma clotting factor VII, red, white and certain renal cells. The body has natural plasmin inhibitors, such as *antiplasmin*. These ensure that widespread destruction of fibrin does not take place.

Blood clotting and the development of thrombosis

Thrombosis is the formation of a clot in a vessel within the cardiovascular system, which relates to or arises from a disease process. There are three factors that increase the likelihood of thrombosis occurring:

1. injury to the vessel wall;
2. altered blood flow;
3. increased likelihood of the blood to clot.

Factor	Name
I	Fibrinogen
II	Prothrombin
III	Tissue factor or thromboplastin
IV	Calcium
V	Proaccelerin (labile factor)
VII	Proconvertin (stable factor)
VIII	Antihaemophilic factor A Antihaemophilic globulin
IX	Antihaemophilic factor B Plasma thromboplastin component Christmas factor
X	Stuart-Prower factor
XI	Plasma thromboplastin antecedent Haemophilia C Rosenthal syndrome
XII	Hageman factor
XIII	Fibrin stabilizing factor Laki-Lorand factor

Table 6.1 Plasma clotting factors

For example, people who have developed fatty plaques, who are physically immobile or who are being treated with certain contraceptives are more at risk of developing thrombosis. Thrombosis can occur in both arteries and veins. In arteries the clot is usually associated with a build up of fatty plaques (atherosclerosis) and has a large platelet component. Veins, in contrast, are usually associated with slow flow of blood through the vessels and there is a large fibrin component. Due to the make-up of the venous thrombosis, the clot has a large jelly-like tail that floats in the vessel. If this breaks off, it becomes what is known as an embolus. This embolus may then lodge in smaller vessels, causing death of tissue.

There are three categories of drugs that affect blood clotting and the formation of thrombosis:

1. drugs that affect fibrin formation;
2. drugs that affect platelet function;
3. drugs that affect dissolving of the clot.

Drugs that act on the clotting cascade

Drugs in this category can be used to manipulate the cascade system when there is a defect in the process of clotting, or when there is an unwanted coagulation taking place.

Fortunately, deficiencies in clotting factors rarely happen. However, two examples need to be mentioned here: haemophilia A, caused by lack of factor VIII and 'Christmas' disease or haemophilia B, caused by lack of factor IX or the 'Christmas' factor (named after Stephen Christmas, the first patient to be diagnosed). These missing factors can be replaced by either giving fresh plasma or giving concentrated preparations of factors VIII and IX. Other problems that lead to an inability of the cascade mechanism to produce clotting are acquired. These tend to be more common in origin and include liver diseases, vitamin K deficiency (especially in neonates) and excessive oral anticoagulants being prescribed. These three situations require the person to be given treatment by administering vitamin K.

Vitamin K

This vitamin is named after 'K' for 'Koagulation' in the German language. It occurs naturally in plants and is essential for the plasma clotting factors we discussed earlier. It is particularly important for formation of factors II, VII, IX and X.

Naturally occurring vitamin K or *phytomenadiole* can be given by mouth or by IV infusion. If it is given orally its absorption will rely on the person's digestive system being normal so that what are known as *bile salts* are being produced and excreted into the duodenum. However, if this is not the case, such as in obstructive jaundice, a synthetic preparation is available that does not require these bile salts in order to be absorbed into the body. This drug is known as *menadiol sodium phosphate*. Vitamin K is used clinically in a range of situations, for example, overdose with warfarin, in babies to prevent haemorrhagic disease and in diseases which cause vitamin K deficiency.

Heparin

Heparin is a complex protein and is found in the liver and mast cells. It is a powerful anticoagulant but is broken down by digestive enzymes; therefore, it is given by IV infusion. Heparin leads to anticoagulation of blood both inside and outside the blood vessels. It works by activating antithrombin III. As you will remember, we discussed the role of this in the section on formation of the fibrin clot. Antithrombin III is a naturally occurring anticoagulant in the body and heparin accelerates its rate of action significantly. This in turn stops the cascade at the thrombin stage, so inhibiting the fibrinogen to fibrin stage of blood clotting from taking place.

Heparin acts immediately following IV administration and its elimination half life is approximately 40 to 90 minutes. In emergency situations, therefore, it is usually given by a bolus dose, followed by a constant rate infusion via a pump mechanism. It is important that the patient is not given too much heparin or they will haemorrhage. A special blood test is performed so that this does not happen. The appropriate blood examination is called an *activated partial thromboplastin time test*. This test will monitor the effects of heparin on blood clotting. Basically, the test measures in seconds how long it takes the blood sample to clot. The dose of heparin is adjusted so that a value of 1.5–2.5 times the normal sample is achieved.

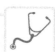

Clinical tip

The obvious main problem with administering heparin is haemorrhage. This often appears as blood in the urine (haematuria) but bleeding from other sites should also be treated seriously. If bleeding does occur, the therapy should be stopped immediately and, if necessary, the patient should be given protamine sulphate which reverses the action of heparin.

A rare complication of heparin is a decrease in the amount of circulating platelets (thrombocytopenia). The patient's platelet count should be ascertained if they remain on the therapy for more than five days. Osteoporosis has been reported in people who have been receiving long-term administration of heparin, although why this occurs is not understood.

Low molecular weight heparins

These are relatively new additions to the anticoagulant drugs available. Basically, they are heparin but broken into smaller parts. This has significant advantages: for example, these drugs are more predictable than their larger cousin, which means that blood tests such as the activated partial thromboplastin time test do not need to be monitored and the dosage does not need to be adjusted. Since this group of drugs can be given satisfactorily by a SC and usually twice-daily route, the need to bring patients into hospital for treatment has been removed. Many of them are treated on an outpatient basis from nurse-led clinics which is far more cost effective.

Low molecular weight heparins can be given to lessen the risk of thrombosis development post-surgery (prophylaxis). The drug is given via the SC route twice a day until the patient is able to mobilize well. It is effective in treating deep vein thrombosis and pulmonary embolism and as the drug does not cross the placental barrier can be used safely in pregnancy. Examples of drugs in this group are Tinzaparin, Enoxaparin, Dalkeparin and Certoparin. Bleeding can occur, but these drugs are less likely than heparin to cause thrombocytopenia.

Enoxaparin

You will come across this medicine under the trade name of Clexane. The medicine in the UK is indicated in six recognized situations, among them stopping thromboembolism post-operatively.

Enoxaparin binds to and accelerates the activity of antithrombin III. By activating antithrombin III, it speeds up the inhibition of coagulation factors Xa (Stuart-Prower) and IIa (prothrombin), where 'a' stands for 'activated'. The anticoagulant effect of enoxaparin can be directly mirrored to its ability to inhibit factor Xa. Factor Xa initiates the conversion of prothrombin to thrombin, so enoxaparin's inhibition of this process results in decreased thrombin and ultimately the prevention of fibrin clot formation.

The usual adult dose to prevent thromboembolism is 40mg subcutaneously once a day. The usual duration of administration is 6 to 11 days; up to 14 days administration has been well tolerated in clinical trials. As a student nurse you will expected to give this medicine and also teach the patient how to administer it to themselves. Enoxaparin should be injected under the skin (SC) usually once or twice a day in the abdomen (at least 50mm from the belly button). It should not be injected into a muscle or vein.

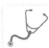

Clinical tip

Before using enoxaparin, check it visually for particles or discoloration. If either is present, do not use the drug. To minimize irritation, change the injection site with each dose. To minimize bruising, do not rub the site after injection.

Mild irritation, pain, bruising, redness or swelling at the injection site may occur and the patient should be reassured that this is not unusual. Inform them that fatigue or fever may also occur and that if these effects persist or worsen they should notify their doctor or pharmacist promptly. Many people using this medication do not have serious side-effects. However it can cause bleeding if its effect on blood clotting proteins is too great. The patient should tell their doctor immediately if any of the following unlikely but serious signs occur: unusual pain, swelling, discomfort, unusual or prolonged bleeding, unusual or 'easy' bruising, dark urine, black stools, severe headache, confusion, vision changes, dizziness, fainting, seizures, weakness and numbness. A very serious allergic reaction to this drug is unlikely.

Hirudin

This anticoagulant is a naturally occurring protein found in the salivary glands of medicinal leeches. Rather than potentiating the effects of antithrombin III, hirudin is a specific inhibitor of thrombin. The problem with this product is the difficulty in extracting commercial amounts. However, it can now be produced by recombinant techniques – a genetically engineered production of the substance to satisfy demands. It is unclear whether this product will replace heparin or the low molecular weight heparins. However, the drug has the advantage of being less likely to trigger immune thrombocytopenia.

Warfarin

It would stand to reason that if vitamin K is so important to the clotting process, any interference with it would result in that process taking longer. This is the basis of the action of the vitamin K antagonist group of anticoagulants, for example, warfarin. The drug blocks the action of vitamin K and so reduces the manufacture of prothrombin and clotting factors VII, IX and X. The onset of action of warfarin takes several days as the plasma factors that have been manufactured prior to commencement of warfarin take time to be eliminated from the body.

Warfarin is given in tablet form as it is easily absorbed by the GI tract. One of the problems with warfarin is that it is strongly attracted to plasma proteins. These proteins normally help maintain the osmotic intravascular pressure. However, as warfarin is bound to these, potential problems occur with stabilizing the dose, treating elderly people and giving other drugs which compete for binding sites on the plasma proteins – for example, aspirin. The peak pharmacological concentration takes approximately 48 hours. The effectiveness of the drug is measured by a blood test known as the *prothrombin time*, now expressed as an international normalized ratio or INR. This laboratory test measures the time it takes for blood to clot and compares it to an average. The higher the INR value, the longer it takes for blood to clot.

Clinical tip

While taking warfarin, patients will have regular blood tests to establish their INR. In a healthy person, you would expect the INR to be 1.0. For patients receiving anticoagulants the INR typically should be between 2.0 and 3.0 for patients who have been diagnosed with atrial fibrillation. Patients who have been fitted with mechanical heart valves should have an INR around 3.0 or 4.0.

Warfarin crosses the placenta and therefore should not be given in the first three months of pregnancy as foetal abnormalities may ensue. Intracranial bleeding in the baby may occur during delivery.

As with heparin, the most obvious side-effect is bleeding. This may be due to deliberate or accidental overdose or to the warfarin interacting with other drugs which leads to an increase in its anticoagulant effect. If bleeding does occur the drug may be withdrawn. The anticoagulant effects may be reversed by giving fresh frozen plasma or vitamin K (phytomenadione) intravenously.

A complication of warfarin is a condition referred to as warfarin necrosis, which occurs as a result of a tendency for the blood to clot. This may seem paradoxical as warfarin is given for its anticoagulant effect, however, this drug, by its vitamin K blocking action, not only affects the plasma coagulation previously outlined but also a naturally occurring blood anticoagulant called protein C. Protein C depends on vitamin K and because this is no longer available cannot be manufactured. The problem occurs because protein C initially decreases at a faster rate than the other coagulation factors. This means that at the commencement of therapy the blood has a tendency to coagulate for a short period.

A variety of disease processes and drugs can modify the action of warfarin. Some potentiate the anticoagulant actions while others lessen the effect of the drug. Liver disease, thyrotoxicosis and fever may all interfere with the natural manufacture by the body of clotting factors. If warfarin is given in these cases an increase in anticoagulation occurs.

Drugs can also lead to exaggerated anticoagulant effects if given in conjunction with warfarin. Drugs such as Cimetidine can reduce the breakdown of warfarin by liver enzymes. NSAIDs compete successfully with warfarin for a place on plasma proteins, therefore leaving more active drugs in the plasma. Antibiotics are another group of drugs that need careful attention before prescribing because broad spectrum antibiotics and some sulfonamides depress the body's natural ability to manufacture vitamin K by intestinal flora.

Anticoagulant effects can also be lessened in certain situations. Hypothyroidism is associated with a slower breakdown of coagulation factors. Foods and commercially produced preparations containing high vitamin K content will reduce the warfarin effect. Also, drugs that cause the enzymes in the liver that break down warfarin to increase, such as Carbamazepine, will have the same effect.

Warfarin is a complex drug that needs to be monitored carefully, and good discharge advice is crucial.

Clinical tip

Many hospitals have advice for patients who receive warfarin, explaining the therapy. All patients should receive a copy of this. It usually details why the person is taking the drug, side-effects, what an INR means and the importance of taking the medication at the same time each day. Advice is also essential regarding some lifestyle changes that need to be made to ensure the patient gets the greatest benefits from taking the drug. Consequently, the patient should receive advice on healthy eating, consumption of alcohol and preventing injury and/or bleeding while taking warfarin. Finally, the patient should have information regarding dental treatment and what to do in the event of an injury or if bleeding takes place. The patient will also be given an anticoagulant card to remind them of the dose they are taking or to be prescribed in the future by either the anticoagulant clinic or the GP.

Future anticoagulant therapy

Rivaroxaban is the first in a new class of drugs known as oral factor Xa (Stuart-Prower) inhibitors. By inhibiting factor Xa, thrombin production and the formation of clots are ultimately inhibited. Currently rivaroxaban is licensed for the prevention of venous thromboembolism (VTE) in adults undergoing elective hip or knee replacement surgery, at a fixed dose of 10mg daily. The obvious beauty of this drug is that it can be given orally.

Rivaroxaban has predictable pharmacokinetics, with little variation of plasma concentration with age, weight, or renal function following a fixed dose. With a fixed dose, a wide therapeutic window, few drug interactions and predictable pharmacodynamics, no routine monitoring of coagulation parameters is required. Rivaroxaban is well absorbed from the gut and maximum inhibition of factor Xa occurs four hours after a dose. The effects last 8–12 hours, but factor Xa activity does not return to normal within 24 hours so once-daily dosing is possible.

Dabigatran is an anticoagulant from the class of direct thrombin inhibitors. It is being studied for various clinical indications and in some cases offers an alternative to warfarin as the preferred orally administered anticoagulant since it does not require frequent blood tests for INR monitoring while offering similar results in terms of efficacy.

Dabigatran etexilate is a pro-drug with no anticoagulant activity; once absorbed, it is rapidly converted by enzymes in the GI tract, blood and liver into dabigatran, a thrombin inhibitor. Although costly, dabigatran etexilate has several potential advantages over warfarin. The pharmacokinetics are quite predictable, simplifying dosing and eliminating the need for frequent blood tests and monitoring. In addition, the drug requires no dietary restrictions and has relatively few drug interactions (at least that are known at this point). Known potential drug interactions are with quinidine, ketoconazole, amiodarone, rifampicin and verapamil. Peak anticoagulation effects occur between half an hour and two hours after ingestion and dabigatran is primarily eliminated by the kidneys.

Antiplatelet drugs

Earlier in this chapter we discussed the importance of the formation of a platelet plug in haemostasis. Drugs that affect this important process have strong therapeutic value. Probably the most common and popular in this category is aspirin.

Aspirin

In the platelet plug discussion we highlighted two important substances that work in opposing ways on the stickiness of blood. These are thromboxane, which increases the stickiness, and prostacyclin which decreases the stickiness. Aspirin alters the fine balance between these two prostaglandins. It reduces both substances in the body but because prostacyclin can be made by endothelial cells and thromboxane levels have to wait between 7 and 10 days for new platelets to be made, prostacyclin levels are improved at the expense of thromboxane. Therefore, an anticoagulant effect is achieved. Aspirin does have a number of serious side-effects but these are limited as it is given at a low dose for its anticoagulant effect. A dose of 75mg daily is sufficient to achieve anticoagulation, in comparison to a dose of 300mg daily which would be prescribed in aspirin's role as an analgesic. Aspirin may be given for a number of conditions, including coronary thrombosis, angina and following transient ischaemic attacks or stroke. A drug by the name of Dipyridamole also prevents platelets sticking together. This drug in combination with aspirin has been shown to be effective in reducing the risk of stroke.

Clopidogrel

This is a fairly new and powerful antiplatelet medicine. You may come across it in your placements, being used for a variety of conditions including coronary artery disease, peripheral vascular disease and cerebrovascular disease.

The drug works by blocking receptor sites on the platelets. This means that when fibrin is formed it cannot stick to the platelet so the plug to block bleeding does not occur as the platelets cannot clump together. It is sometimes used alongside aspirin.

Clopidogrel can be given orally and is normally prescribed at 75mg once per day. It is a pro-drug activated by the liver when it first passes through. Once the drug has been activated its elimination half life is eight hours. The drug reaches a peak level in the blood after one hour.

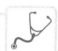

> **Clinical tip**
>
> Haemorrhage is by far the most common side-effect of this class of drug. You should ask the patient to report any unusual bleeding or bruising. Side-effects can also include neutropenia (low level of a type of white blood cell called a neutrophil in the bloodstream). Therefore you should encourage the patient to contact their doctor if they experience fever, signs of infection or extreme tiredness.

Abciximab

As described earlier the final part of the platelet plug formation is the depositing of substances on platelets that allows fibrin strands to anchor to them. Abciximab interferes with this process. It is given intravenously and usually only indicated in high risk patients undergoing certain invasive procedures such as coronary angioplasty. Because of its risk of causing an immune response its use is usually limited to one dose only.

Fibrinolytic drugs

These drugs mimic the body's own ability to dissolve blood clots. A number of drugs are used in practice that dissolve clots in order to allow free passage of blood back to an area that has been starved of blood (i.e. that is ischaemic). The main use is in patients who have had acute myocardial infarction following blockages of the coronary artery.

Clinical tip

Often in practice you will hear people refer to fibrinolytic drugs as 'clot busters'.

Clinical tip

The main risk with streptokinase is the risk of haemorrhage. This normally occurs near the injection site and sites of recent trauma. You must constantly monitor the site of administration and document any untoward signs and symptoms. It is contraindicated in patients in whom it may cause bleeding — for example, patients with peptic ulcers. Therefore it is important to ask the patient about their past medical history before administration of this drug.

Streptokinase

This drug is used to dissolve the fibrin of blood clots, especially those that occur in the heart and lungs. Acute myocardial infarction results from blockage of a coronary artery, which results in an area of heart muscle being deprived of blood. Streptokinase is used in breaking down such clots in the coronary vessels.

The drug triggers the plasma protein plasminogen to liberate plasmin, which breaks down fibrin, so dissolving the clot. The drug is extracted from bacteria called *haemolytic streptococci*. It has a short half life of less than 20 minutes and is therefore given by continuous IV infusion. Most people will have developed antibodies to streptococcal proteins, so often a large bolus dose is used to start therapy, followed by a maintenance infusion. As antibodies form against the streptococcal proteins it is usually best not to give another treatment with the drug until a year has elapsed. Also, due to the body's immune response, other drugs, such as chlorphenamine or hydrocortisone, may be given to reduce any allergic response.

Alteplase

This drug is derived from human tissue plasminogen activator. Therefore, it directly converts plasminogen to plasmin. It binds strongly with fibrin and digests clots in coronary arteries at least as well if not better than streptokinase. It has the advantages of not causing immune responses and, having a greater attraction to fibrin-bound plasminogen rather than circulating plasma fibrinogen, is said to be 'clot selective'. As with streptokinase, the drug has a short half life and is therefore given by IV infusion. Even though alteplase is less likely to cause bleeding, it is contraindicated in pregnancy, uncontrolled hypertension, haemorrhagic cerebrovascular disease and active internal bleeding. If bleeding occurs it can be treated with tranexamic acid. This stops plasminogen activation and therefore prevents clots dissolving. The patient may also be given fresh plasma or coagulation factors.

Case study

Olek Krupa is a 65-year-old widower. He has his own business, which is a roofing company.
His aim is to retire in a couple of years' time so he is increasingly leaving his sons to manage the business while he enjoys more golfing holidays. He lives on his own but has a wide circle of friends. He enjoys watching football and having a few pints at his local pub. He does this on a few nights or afternoons in the week. He recently visited his GP for a check-up but prior to this had not seen his doctor for a number of years. He was found to have high blood pressure, be overweight and to have a heart condition for which the GP prescribed aspirin. Further to this, he was referred to his local cardiologist, who recommended that he stop the aspirin in favour of commencing warfarin. What advice would you give to Mr Krupa with regard to his warfarin therapy?

Key learning points

Introduction

➢ Blood clotting is a normal homeostatic mechanism.
➢ Haemostasis is divided into four processes: constriction of blood vessel, formation of platelet plug, formation of fibrin clot and dissolving of the clot.
➢ Constriction of the vessel reduces blood flow.
➢ Constriction allows clotting factors to come into contact with the damaged vessels.
➢ Formation of a platelet plug begins with exposure to collagen and elastin fibres.
➢ Platelets release thromboxane.
➢ The formation of a fibrin clot is a complex chain reaction triggered in two ways: extrinsically and intrinsically.
➢ The clot dissolves more slowly than it was built.
➢ Fibrin is dissolved by plasmin.

Blood clotting and the development of thrombosis

➢ Injury to vessels, altered blood flow and increased likelihood of clotting all influence the risk of thrombosis.
➢ Vitamin K naturally occurs in plants.
➢ It is essential for the synthesis of plasma clotting factors.
➢ Vitamin K is given for overdose of warfarin and in haemorrhagic disease of the newborn.

Heparin

➢ Heparin is a complex protein which cannot be given orally.
➢ It works by activating antithrombin III.
➢ It stops the clotting cascade at the thrombin stage.
➢ Activated partial thromboplastin time test is used to measure efficacy.
➢ Low molecular weight heparins are more predictable.
➢ They are given subcutaneously twice daily.
➢ Examples are tinzaparin and exoxaparin.

Enoxaparin

➢ Enoxaparin binds to and accelerates the activity of antithrombin III.
➢ Dose to prevent thromboembolism is 40 mg subcutaneously once a day.
➢ The usual duration of administration is 6 to 11 days, up to 14 days.
➢ To minimize irritation, change the injection site with each dose.
➢ To minimize bruising, do not rub the injection site following administration.
➢ The patient should tell their doctor immediately if signs of bleeding occur.

→

Warfarin

➢ Warfarin is a vitamin K antagonist.
➢ It reduces the manufacture of a range of clotting factors.
➢ It takes several days to achieve its effects.
➢ It is highly protein bound.
➢ It is measured by the INR.
➢ Can cross placental barrier.
➢ Haemorrhage is a major side-effect.
➢ A number of disease processes and other drugs can potentiate or inhibit its action.
➢ Patients need detailed discharge advice.

Future anticoagulant therapy

➢ Rivaroxaban is the first oral factor Xa (Stuart-Prower) inhibitor.
➢ Dabigatran is an option for primary prevention of venous thromboembolic event.

Aspirin

➢ Aspirin alters the fine balance between thromboxane and prostacyclin.
➢ It is given in low dosages to limit side-effects.
➢ It is suitable for a number of conditions (e.g. coronary thrombosis).

Clopidogrel

➢ Stops fibrin attaching to platelets.
➢ Often given alongside low dose aspirin.
➢ Haemorrhage is a common side-effect.

Streptokinase

➢ Dissolves fibrin.
➢ Liberates plasmin from plasminogen.
➢ One treatment is given per year.
➢ Risk of haemorrhage.

Alteplase

➢ Converts plasminogen to plasmin.
➢ Does not cause immune response like streptokinase.
➢ Has to be given intravenously.
➢ Contraindicated in pregnancy, haemorrhagic cerebrovascular disease and internal bleeding.

Calculations

1 A doctor orders a patient to have 25,000 international units (iu) of heparin which is to be given intravenously. On the ward you only have 5,000iu of heparin in 1ml. How many ml of heparin would you give?

2 A patient has been prescribed 300mg of aspirin. You have 75mg tablets. How many would you need to administer?

3 The dose of tinzaparin for the treatment of deep vein thrombosis is 175 units per kg. The injection is 20,000 units per ml. What dose would be required to treat a 60kg patient?

4 A doctor orders heparin 9,000iu to be given subcutaneously twice daily. The ward stock only consists of 10,000iu per ml. How many ml of heparin would you give?

5 Warfarin is available as 0.5mg, 1mg, 3mg and 5mg tablets. You need to administer a 7mg dose. What is the least number of tablets you can give?

6 20,000iu of heparin is added to 500ml of 0.9 per cent saline. The dose prescribed is 200iu per hour. Calculate the rate of the infusion in ml per hour.

7 You need to give 1mg of vitamin K orally. How many ml of a 10mg per ml vitamin K injection would you give?

8 You have been asked to prepare a heparin syringe for intravenous infusion; 40ml of solution is required, containing 500 units of heparin per ml. The heparin ampoules stocked on the ward contain 5000 units per ml. What volume of heparin and saline would be required to prepare the syringe?

9 You have a syringe of enoxaparin containing 150 mg per ml. How much is required to give a 90kg man a dose of 1.5mg per kg?

10 An anaesthetist prescribes a patient dalteparin sodium 2500iu two hours prior to surgery, 2500iu four to eight hours post-surgery and 5000iu daily for 5–10 days post-operative. How many ml from a vial containing 10,000iu per ml should be administered:

   a) Prior to surgery?
   b) After surgery?
   c) The following day after surgery?

For further assistance with calculations, please see Meriel Hutton's *Essential Calculation Skills for Nurses, Midwives and Healthcare Practitioners* (Open University Press 2009).

Multiple choice questions

Try answering these multiple choice questions to test what you have learned from reading this chapter. You can check your answers on page 201.

1 Haemophilia A is caused by a lack of which clotting factor?

a) Factor X

←

b) Factor VII
c) Factor VIII
d) Factor III

2 Where in the body is heparin normally manufactured?

a) Liver
b) Kidney
c) Spleen
d) Pancreas

3 What substance does heparin activate in order to produce its anticoagulant effect?

a) Antithrombin
b) Thromboxane
c) Prostacyclin
d) Fibrinogen

4 What drug reverses the effects of heparin?

a) Warfarin
b) Aspirin
c) Vitamin K
d) Protamine sulphate

5 How does warfarin work?

a) Decreases the amount of circulating platelets
b) Increases the amount of antithrombin
c) Antagonizes vitamin K
d) Increases the amount of prostacyclin

6 Which of the following drugs is a low molecular weight heparin?

a) Clopidogrel
b) Tinzaparin
c) Dipyridamole
d) Hirudin

7 What blood test is used to measure the effectiveness of warfarin?

a) International normalized ratio
b) International notifiable ratio
c) Internal negative report
d) Integrated notice of randomization

→

←

8 Aspirin has an effect on the balance of which two substances?

a) Thromboxane and fibrinogen
b) Prostacyclin and calcium
c) Thromboxane and prostacyclin
d) Antithrombin and thrombin

9 Which of the following is a fibrinolytic medicine?

a) Beconase
b) Lipase
c) Alteplase
d) Mono amine oxidase

10 The main mode of action of fibrinolytic drugs is

a) Increase the amount of vitamin K
b) Decrease the amount of platelets
c) Decrease the amount of plasmin
d) Increase the amount of plasmin

Recommended further reading

Beckwith, S. and Franklin, P. (2007) *Oxford Handbook of Nurse Prescribing*. Oxford: Oxford University Press.

Brenner, G.M. and Stevens, C.W. (2006) *Pharmacology*, 2nd edn. Philadelphia, PA: Saunders Elsevier.

Casey, G. (2003) Continuing professional development: haemostasis, anticoagulants and fibrinolysis, *Nursing Standard*, 18: 45–51.

Clayton, B.D. (2009) *Basic Pharmacology for Nurses*, 15th edn. St Louis, MO: Mosby Elsevier.

Coben, D. and Atere-Roberts, E. (2005) *Calculations for Nursing and Healthcare*, 2nd edn. Basingstoke: Palgrave Macmillan.

Downie, G., Mackenzie, J. and Williams, A. (2007) *Pharmacology and Medicines Management for Nurses*, 4th edn. Edinburgh: Churchill Livingstone.

Gallagher, D. and Rix, E. (2006) Understanding the implications of oral anticoagulation therapy, *Nursing Times*, 102: 30–2.

Gatford, J.D. and Phillips, N. (2006) *Nursing Calculations*, 7th edn. Edinburgh: Churchill Livingstone Elsevier.

Karch, A.M. (2008) *Focus on Nursing Pharmacology*, 4th edn. Philadelphia, PA: Lippincott Williams & Wilkins.

Lake, R. and Jordan, S. (2005) Prescription drugs: uses and effects, anticoagulants, *Nursing Standard*, 19(19).

Lapham, R. and Agar, H. (2003) *Drug Calculations for Nurses: A Step-by-step Approach*, 2nd edn. London: Arnold.

NICE (National Institute for Health and Clinical Excellence) (2006) *Clinical Guideline 36: Atrial Fibrillation*. London: NICE.

NICE (National Institute for Health and Clinical Excellence) (2007) *Clinical Guideline 48: Secondary Prevention of Myocardial Infarction*. London: NICE.

NICE (National Institute for Health and Clinical Excellence) (2008) *Technology Appraisal TA 157: Dabigatran Etexilate for the Prevention of Venous Thromboembolism After Hip or Knee Replacement Surgery in Adults*. London: NICE.

NICE (National Institute for Health and Clinical Excellence) (2009) *Technology Appraisal TA 170: Rivaroxaban for the Prevention of Venous Thromboembolism*. London: NICE.

Simonson, T., Aarbakke, J., Kay, I., Coleman, I., Sinnott, P. and Lyssa, R. (2006) *Illustrated Pharmacology for Nurses*. London: Hodder Arnold.

Trounce, J. (2000) *Clinical Pharmacology for Nurses*, 16th edn. New York: Churchill Livingstone.

Drugs used in chronic conditions

7

Chapter contents

Learning objectives
Introduction
Asthma
  Pathological changes in asthma
  Asthma in children
Drugs used in treating asthma
  Beta 2 adrenoreceptor agonists
  Methylxanthines
  Muscarinic receptor antagonists
  Ipratropium
  Inhaled corticosteroids
  Cromoglicate
Chronic obstructive pulmonary disease
Diabetes
Medicine management of diabetes
  Insulin
    Treatment with insulin
    Short-acting insulins
    Intermediate insulins
    Long-acting insulins
    Side-effects
    Insulin pumps
  Oral hypoglycaemic agents
    Metformin
    Sulfonylureas
    Meglitinides
    Thiazolidinediones (glitazones)

  Alpha-glucosidase inhibitors
Hypertension
  Thiazide diuretics
  Beta-adrenoreceptor antagonists
  Angiotensin-converting enzyme inhibitors
  Calcium antagonists
  Alpha-adrenoreceptor antagonists
Parkinson's disease
  Levodopa
  Selegiline
  Dopamine receptor agonists
  Acetylcholine antagonists
Epilepsy
  Partial seizures
  Generalized seizures
  Inhibition of sodium channel function
    Phenytoin
  Inhibition of calcium channels
    Ethosuximide
  Enhancement of GABA action
    Sodium valproate
    Vigabatrin
Case studies
Key learning points
Calculations
Multiple choice questions
Recommended further reading

Learning objectives

After studying this chapter you should be able to:

● Describe the basic pathology involved in asthma, diabetes, hypertension, Parkinson's disease and epilepsy.
● Explain the mode of action of medicines used in treating these conditions.
● Demonstrate an understanding of the unwanted effects of medicines used in treating these conditions.
● Discuss the correct technique involved when teaching a person to use an inhaler.
● Demonstrate an understanding of the links between the pharmacology of therapies used in treating asthma, diabetes, hypertension, Parkinson's disease and epilepsy and the care given by the health practitioner.
● Correctly solve a number of drug calculations with regard to medicines used in the treatment of these conditions.

Introduction

A large number of chronic diseases are brought about by demographic, environmental and lifestyle changes. Common conditions include asthma, diabetes, hypertension, Parkinson's disease and epilepsy. This chapter will focus on the drug management of each of these conditions. The chapter is only introductory and is not intended as comprehensive coverage of all chronic conditions and their pharmaceutical management.

Asthma

Asthma is the leading chronic disease in developed countries and its incidence is increasing. The condition is brought on by a reversible obstruction of the airways which in turn causes the individual to become breathless and start to cough or wheeze. Asthma may be described as being acute or chronic. Severe acute asthma (known as *status asthmaticus*) is not reversed very easily and, as a result, continues to be fatal and requires prompt treatment. Chronic asthma usually has an intermittent pattern of breathlessness (dyspnoea), coughing and wheezing.

In acute asthma the main reason for obstruction of the airways is *bronchoconstriction* caused by a substance called histamine. Further significant obstruction of the airways is brought about by inflammatory changes in the mucosa which cause an increase in mucous production, more epithelial cells being shed and swelling of the tissues within the respiratory passages.

Asthma symptoms are thought to be caused by what doctors describe as hyper-reactivity or hyper-responsiveness of the cells lining the air passages. It seems that bronchiolar tissue in certain individuals is more sensitive to certain trigger factors than other people in the general population. Trigger factors include irritant chemicals, exposure to foreign proteins called allergens, and cold air.

Numerous cells and chemicals play a part in the changes that take place in the tissues of a person who suffers from asthma. We will now consider these changes in order to provide an understanding of how drugs used in this condition work.

Pathological changes in asthma

The changes in the respiratory system that bring about asthma are initiated by an allergic reaction. The trigger factor stimulates the body's immune response and as part of this the body produces a type of white cell called a *B-lymphocyte*. Some of these B-lymphocytes mature into a type of cell called a *plasma cell*. These cells produce a chemical called *immunoglobulin E* which is a type of antibody. These antibodies in turn attach themselves to a type of tissue cell called a *mast cell*.

These mast cells are now stimulated to produce a substance called histamine. Histamine is a potent constrictor of the muscles in the air passages, causing them to become narrowed. This is called *bronchoconstriction*. Histamine also causes local blood vessels to dilate and become more permeable so that other inflammatory cells in the plasma can move into the tissues. Not only does histamine cause constriction of bronchial smooth muscle, it also leads to swelling of the tissues.

Another specific group of white cells thought to be involved in asthma are the *eosinophils*. This group of cells are implicated in the inflammatory response by releasing a range of chemicals that contribute to the contraction of bronchial smooth muscle, permeability of small blood vessels and excessive secretion of mucous. It is also suggested that the eosinophils produce chemicals that have a toxic effect on the epithelial lining of the airways and are responsible for the greater amount of epithelial shedding associated with this condition.

Macrophages are a type of bacteria-engulfing cell or phagocyte which are protective in function. However, in asthma these cells are responsible for releasing a group of substances called *prostaglandins* and platelet-activating factors which sustain the bronchial hyperactivity. This is thought to occur by increasing mucosal oedema, facilitating the number of eosinophils in the airway tissues.

The swelling of the local tissues from oedema is compounded by extra mucous production. Mucous is part of our general defence strategy in that it provides us with a mechanism to trap particles and bacteria and clear them from the upper respiratory tract. However, in asthma the size of the bronchial glands and goblet cells is increased and they subsequently produce large amounts of mucous which is thickened by cell debris from the epithelial shedding. The cilia that normally waft debris towards the pharynx also have their capability curtailed, contributing to the overall obstruction of the person's air passages.

Asthma in children

Asthma is the leading cause of chronic illness in children. It affects as many as 15 per cent of children in the UK and, for unknown reasons, is steadily increasing. It can begin at any age, but most children have their first symptoms by age 5. Children still die from asthma – there were 27 recorded deaths in 2005 – and there is still significant disability associated with the disease, particularly severe childhood asthma, despite pharmacological advances.

There are many risk factors for developing childhood asthma, including:

- presence of allergies;
- family history of asthma and/or allergies;
- frequent respiratory infections;
- low birth weight;
- exposure to tobacco smoke before and/or after birth;
- being male;
- being black;
- obesity;
- being raised in a low-income environment.

No one really knows why more and more children are developing asthma. Some experts suggest that children are being exposed to more and more allergens such as dust, air pollution and second-hand smoke. These factors are all triggers of asthma. Others suspect that children are not exposed to enough childhood illnesses to build up their immune system, meaning that the body fails to make enough protective antibodies. Still others suggest that decreasing rates of breastfeeding have prevented important substances of the immune system from being passed on to babies.

Diagnosis of asthma in children is difficult because of the complex nature of the disorder in the young. In an adult a wheeze is a very important sign in the diagnosis of asthma, however in children there are many different causes of wheeze. In addition, children younger than five are generally unable to perform pulmonary function tests with the result that doctors rely heavily on history, symptoms and examination in making a diagnosis.

Most asthma medications that are given to adults and older children can also safely be prescribed to toddlers and younger children. Drugs that are approved for younger children are given in doses adjusted for their age and weight. Specifically, children of 4 years and up may be prescribed the asthma inhaler seretide. This treats both airway inflammation and bronchoconstriction. In the case of inhaled drugs, a different delivery device based on the child's age and ability may be required because many children are not able to coordinate their breathing well enough to use a standard inhaler.

Clinical tip

You will probably be asked to give a child asthma medications using a nebulizer while on placement. A nebulizer delivers asthma drugs, usually bronchodilators, by changing them from a liquid to a mist. The child gets the drug by breathing it in through a facemask. These breathing treatments usually take about 10–15 minutes and are given several times a day. Children may be able to use a metered dose inhaler (MDI) with a spacer. A spacer is a chamber that attaches to the MDI and holds the burst of medication.

Drugs used in treating asthma

There are two basic drug groups given to patients who have asthma: *bronchodilators* and *anti-inflammatory agents*. They are not mutually exclusive – i.e. some bronchodilators may have an effect on inflammatory cells. Bronchodilators are the first group of drugs that we will focus upon.

Beta 2 adrenoreceptor agonists

These drugs are referred to as *bronchodilators*. They open the air passages by directly activating beta receptors, relaxing the smooth muscle in the walls of the bronchioles. This allows a more normal movement of air between the atmosphere and the alveoli. This group of drugs is available in both short- and long-acting forms. An example of a short-acting form in this class is salbutamol.

Clinical tip

Beta 2 adrenoreceptor agonists are often referred to as 'rescue remedies' because they ease the difficult breathing (dyspnoea), shortness of breath and wheezing associated with an asthma attack. Generally, these drugs have a short period of action.

Most short-acting beta 2 agonists are available as aerosols to inhale by mouth several times a day. Most are also available as solutions that can be used with a special apparatus called a *nebulizer*. The maximum effect occurs within 30 minutes and the duration of action is between four and six hours. The patient is usually prescribed the drug on a 'prn' (*pro re nata* – as required) basis.

Clinical tip

The longer-acting drugs in this class are often called 'controllers' because they help people with moderate to severe asthma control their symptoms. The effects of these drugs are longer-lasting at around 12 hours. An example of a drug in this class is salmeterol.

These medications are also available as dry powders, administered by inhalation. However, they are not prescribed on a prn basis but are taken regularly, such as twice a day. Sometimes you may find this type of drug being used alongside a glucocorticoid preparation.

Beta 2 adrenoreceptor agonists do not control the inflammatory response in asthma and if a patient is finding it difficult to control their symptoms by using this class of drug a corticosteroid preparation may be added. The most common side-effect of beta 2 adrenoreceptor agonists is tremor.

Methylxanthines

The drug from this family most commonly employed in the clinical setting is theophylline, which works as a bronchodilator by relaxing the bronchial smooth muscle. Several mechanisms of action have been proposed but it is still unclear how this drug produces its effects. Recently theophylline has also been shown to have some anti-inflammatory activity, especially with regard to mast cell activity. Theophylline is a useful drug in that it produces bronchial dilation so reducing the symptoms of chronic asthma, reducing the dosage of oral corticosteroids and reducing the requirement for symptomatic use of beta 2 adrenoreceptor agonists.

The drug is well absorbed from the GI tract and therefore can be given orally. Peak levels are achieved within one to two hours. However, if given with food, this will take longer. The drug has a relatively short half life and therefore you will come across a variety of sustained release preparations.

The drug is metabolized in the liver by a group of enzymes called *cytochrome P450*. Therefore, if the patient is taking other drugs using the same enzyme system, theophylline will accumulate. Two examples of drugs that might cause this interaction are erythromycin and ciprofloxacin.

Theophylline is used both in chronic asthma and chronic obstructive pulmonary disease (COPD, see p. 121) and as an emergency treatment in acute severe asthma. Despite its effectiveness it is not used as a first-line treatment but rather a third- or fourth-line option. One of the factors that limits its use is the high incidence of side-effects within its therapeutic range and narrow therapeutic index. As the plasma levels of the drug increase, so do the side-effects and concordance with this drug can be poor because of these side-effects. Theophylline has a stimulant effect on the central nervous system causing increased alertness, and can interfere with sleep. The drug also stimulates the cardiovascular system: the heart rate increases as does the force of contraction and thereby the patient's blood pressure. Indigestion is also a common side-effect, probably due to the drug increasing gastric secretion and relax-ation of the cardiac sphincter, therefore leading to reflux.

Deaths associated with theophylline have been reported and are due to the serious cardiovascular side-effect of dysrhythmia. Seizures are also a further life-threatening side-effect and can occur in concentrations only just above the therapeutic level.

Muscarinic receptor antagonists

The parasympathetic nervous system causes bronchoconstriction; therefore, if these effects on the bronchioles of the lungs were blocked dilatation would take place. This is the basic premise of this group of drugs. The compounds are used mainly in asthma, chronic bronchitis and COPD.

Ipratropium

This medicine comes as a solution to inhale by mouth, either as an aerosol or in a nebulizer. The aerosol is usually prescribed four times a day. The bronchodilator effect begins after approximately 45 minutes and lasts for about three to five hours. This drug can cause side-effects ranging from leaving an unpleasant taste in the mouth and/or a dry mouth to rashes, hoarseness and chest pain.

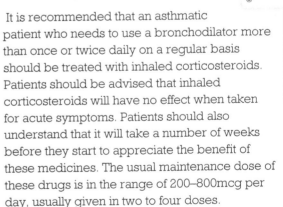

Clinical tip

It is recommended that an asthmatic patient who needs to use a bronchodilator more than once or twice daily on a regular basis should be treated with inhaled corticosteroids. Patients should be advised that inhaled corticosteroids will have no effect when taken for acute symptoms. Patients should also understand that it will take a number of weeks before they start to appreciate the benefit of these medicines. The usual maintenance dose of these drugs is in the range of 200–800mcg per day, usually given in two to four doses.

Inhaled corticosteroids

Glucocorticoids are dealt with in more detail in Chapter 5. They do not bring about bronchodilatation and are not given as an immediate response to the trigger factor. However, inhaled *corticosteroids* are now a regular therapy in asthma management. Two drugs commonly used are beclometasone dipropionate and budesonide. Both have anti-inflammatory and immunosuppressive activity. When inhaled they prevent the production of a chemical called *arachidonic acid* which in turn leads to the reduced formation of prostaglandins and leucotrienes, reducing the inflammatory response (see Chapter 5). Both drugs when taken regularly reduce the frequency of 'rescue' bronchodilator intake.

Inhaled corticosteroids are now preferred to oral steroids because of the reduced incidence of side-effects. However, side-effects do still occur but are usually only local in nature, for example sore and dry throat, and occasionally patients may develop oral thrush (candidiasis).

Clinical tip

Candidiasis can be prevented to some extent by rinsing the mouth after inhaling the drug or using a special device called a spacer which reduces the deposits of the drug in the tissues of the mouth and throat. The patient may have to be treated with antifungal lozenges.

Clinical tip

Inhaler technique

As inhaled medicines are so important in the management of asthma it is equally important that nurses educate their patients in a systematic manner.

1. Get the patient to hold the inhaler with the clear end pointing upwards. Place the metal canister inside the clear end, ensuring that it is fully and firmly in place and that the canister is at room temperature.

2. Remove the protective dust cap from the end of the mouthpiece. If the cap was not placed on the mouthpiece, check the mouthpiece for dirt or other objects.

3. If the patient is using the inhaler for the first time or has not used it in the last three days, get them to prime it by pressing down on the canister to release two sprays into the air, away from their face. Ensure they do not spray the medication into their eyes.

4. Ask the patient to breathe out as completely as possible through their mouth, then to hold the inhaler between the thumb and the next two fingers with the mouthpiece at the bottom and facing them. The patient should then place the open end of the mouthpiece into their mouth and avoid covering the drug outlet piece with their tongue. The patient should close their lips tightly around the mouthpiece and close their eyes.

5. The patient should now breathe in slowly and deeply through the mouthpiece at the same time pressing down firmly on the top of the canister.

6. The patient should hold their breath for a count of 10, then remove the inhaler and breathe out slowly.

7. If the patient is to take another dose, ask them to wait for approximately 15 seconds and then repeat steps 4–6.

8. Finally ask the patient to replace the protective cap on the inhaler.

More serious local side-effects are hoarseness and changes of the voice (dysphonia). General or systemic side-effects are seen in high dosages. Beclometasone may cause weakening of bone (osteoporosis), while other side-effects may include increased bruising and thinning of the skin (dermal thinning).

Cromoglicate

This medicine is not a bronchodilator, however if given prior to an asthmatic attack it prevents the immediate and later bronchoconstrictive reactions to inhaled allergens by stopping the release of mediators such as histamine from mast cells. It is thought that this medicine blocks calcium channels from opening in the mast cells. As calcium is blocked from entering the cells, so in turn is the release of inflammatory mediators. However, its exact mode of action is still not known.

Cromoglicate is given by inhaler, initially two puffs four times daily. For protection against bronchospasm caused by exercise the medicine should be used 15 to 30 minutes beforehand. If adequate response to the medicine is obtained then the dose may be reduced to two to six puffs daily.

The most frequently reported adverse reactions are throat irritation or dryness, a bad taste in the mouth, coughing, wheezing and nausea. Severe anaphylaxis and bronchospasm can occur but are fortunately rare.

Chronic obstructive pulmonary disease

COPD is a general term which includes the conditions chronic bronchitis and emphysema. COPD is the preferred term, but you may also hear it called 'chronic obstructive airways disease' (COAD). Chronic bronchitis and emphysema commonly occur alongside each other, leading to the airways becoming narrowed and a limitation of the flow of air to and from the lungs, causing shortness of breath. In clinical practice, COPD is defined by its characteristically low airflow in lung function tests. In contrast to asthma, this limitation is poorly reversible and usually gets progressively worse over

time. In England, approximately 1 person in 59 is diagnosed with COPD at some point in their lives.

The most common cause of COPD is smoking. Once you give up smoking, you gradually reduce the chances of suffering from COPD, and you slow down its progress if you already have it. Occupational factors, such as coal dust and some inherited problems can also cause COPD. Whether pollution is a factor is under investigation.

A productive cough is usually the first symptom to develop, meaning that the patient produces sputum (phlegm). This cough tends to come and go at first, and then gradually becomes more persistent (chronic). The patient may actually refer to this cough as being a 'smoker's cough' in the early stages of the disease. When breathlessness begins, people often become more concerned.

Breathlessness and a wheeze may at first occur only when the person is exerting themselves, such as when they climb the stairs. The symptoms become gradually worse over the years especially if the person continue to smoke. Difficulty with breathing may eventually become quite distressing.

Chest infections are more common in a person who has COPD. A sudden worsening of symptoms (such as when the patient has an infection) is called an *exacerbation*. Wheezing with a cough and breathlessness become worse than usual and the patient may cough up more sputum than normal. Such infections can be caused by bacteria *or* viruses. Bacteria (which can be killed using antibiotics) cause about one in two or three exacerbations of COPD. Viruses (not killed with antibiotics) such as the common cold virus may also be responsible for up to one in three exacerbations.

Stopping smoking is the most important treatment and no other may be needed if the disease is at an early stage and the symptoms are mild. If symptoms become troublesome, one or more of the following treatments may be advised (treatments do not *cure* COPD but they can ease the symptoms). As a general rule, a trial of one to three months of a treatment will give an indication as to whether it is helpful or not. The main treatments are medications in powdered form given via inhalers.

Box 7.1 Management of asthma for children over 5 into adulthood

Steps	Child key	Adult key
1 – Mild intermittent asthma	Inhaled short-acting beta 2 agonist as required	Inhaled short-acting beta 2 agonist as required
2 – Regular preventer therapy	Add inhaled steroid 200–400mcg per day	Add inhaled steroid 200–800mcg per day
3 – Initial add-on therapy	Add inhaled long-acting beta 2 agonist Assess the control of the asthma	Add inhaled long-acting beta 2 agonist Assess the control of the asthma
4 – Persistent poor control	Increase the inhaled steroid up to 800mcg per day	Consider trials of increasing inhaled steroid up to 2000mcg per day. Add a fourth drug (e.g. slow release theophylline)
5 – Continuous or frequent use of steroids	Use daily steroid tablet	Use daily steroid tablet

Based on the *British Thoracic Society Guidelines* 2008

Drugs that may be considered in treating people diagnosed with COPD are beta-agonists, muscarinic receptor antagonists and the methylanthine drug theophylline (see 'Drugs used in treating asthma' p. 118). During acute exacerbations of the disease antibiotics and steroid medicines will normally be added.

Diabetes

Diabetes mellitus is a chronic disease of metabolism caused by either an insufficient production of insulin in the body or an insufficient effect of insulin in the peripheral tissues. The main problems stem from a wide fluctuation in the range of blood glucose levels which leads to a number of short- and long-term difficulties for the individual. There are two main forms of diabetes: type I and type II.

In type I diabetes the body produces little or no insulin in cells contained in the pancreas and known as the 'Islets of Langerhans' or the beta cells. The pancreas is a specialized gland that lies just behind the stomach. Its functions range from

regulating the amount of sugar (glucose) you have in your blood to producing enzymes that help break down and digest proteins, carbohydrates and fats. It is thought that the beta cells in the pancreas are destroyed by the body's own immune response: hence diabetes is an autoimmune disease. Someone with type I diabetes will be required to take insulin for the rest of their lives.

Clinical tip

Sometimes professionals will refer to type I diabetes as 'juvenile' because it usually starts before the age of 40 and is most common in the teenage years.

In type II diabetes the beta cells may produce small amounts of insulin but not enough to control the levels of glucose in the plasma. In addition, the cells of the body, and particularly in the periphery, cannot utilize insulin properly. This means that glucose is not allowed to enter peripheral cells, so increasing the glucose levels in the plasma. This type of diabetes is linked to the problem of obesity.

Clinical tip

Sometimes you will hear people refer to type II diabetes as 'maturity onset' as it occurs in people over the age of 40.

It is estimated that approximately 2 million people in the UK are currently being treated for type II diabetes. However, researchers suggest that there are as many people who are under-diagnosed. The risk of this type of diabetes is also higher if it runs in the family or if the patient is overweight. From this perspective, it is clear that prevention of obesity will also lead to prevention of type II diabetes.

Without treatment, the main symptoms of diabetes can be divided into two major areas: acute symptoms and chronic complications. There are a number of symptoms that could be referred to as 'classic'. These are excessive thirst (polydypsia), producing lots of urine necessitating many trips to the toilet (polyuria), blurring of vision, tiredness and weight loss due to muscle wasting (loss of muscle mass).

The chronic complications of diabetes are caused by long-term raised glucose levels in the body. This leads to damage, particularly to blood vessels and peripheral nerves.

Clinical tip

'Macrovascular disease' refers to damage to the larger blood vessels and results in coronary heart disease or peripheral vascular disease. 'Microvascular disease' refers to damage to smaller vessels, resulting in eye problems (retinopathy) and kidney damage (nephropathy). Damage to the outside of the nerves (the nerve sheaths) is also a problematic complication. This process is referred to as 'neuropathy'.

Medicine management of diabetes

The overall aim of the treatment of diabetes is to maintain blood glucose levels within the normal range (normoglycaemia). This will relieve the acute symptoms and should minimize the impact of chronic complications on the individual. In reality, achieving normoglycaemia is very difficult and drug treatments are aimed at an individual level. An increase in exercise and cessation of smoking are advisable in order to reduce high blood pressure (hypertension) and high fat content in the blood (hyperlipidaemia). These measures have been shown to reduce the risk of long-term complications of this disease. However, the most important key to treatment of diabetes is diet. This can be used alone or can be combined with the use of insulin or other oral hypoglycaemic agents.

Insulin

The hormone insulin is released in the body as a direct response to a raised blood glucose level. Insulin is released directly into the blood and stimulates the uptake of glucose; it is the key that allows glucose to enter cells, and without it the door remains locked and glucose builds up in the blood. Insulin also promotes conversion of glucose to a substance called *glycogen*, which allows the body to store glucose for periods when the person is not eating but still requires glucose for bodily functions.

Insulin also limits the amount of fat breakdown in the body, a process called *lypolysis*. Triglycerides (large fat molecules) which are normally stored in your fatty (adipose) tissue are broken down into their constituent fatty acids and glycerol. These are then transported to the liver where they are used to fuel certain metabolic pathways. As insulin is either missing or low in quantity in diabetes these metabolic pathways soon become saturated, resulting in the production by the body of acidic compounds such as ketone bodies and acetate.

Treatment with insulin

At one time insulin was extracted from the pancreas of cattle (bovine insulin) or pigs (porcine

Box 7.2 The two types of diabetes

	Type I	Type II
Other names	Juvenile onset diabetes Insulin-dependent diabetes (IDDM)	Maturity onset diabetes. Non-insulin dependent diabetes (NIDDM)
Description	Little or no insulin produced by the pancreas; insulin is required to sustain life, therefore the individual requires daily insulin in order to survive	Pancreas doesn't make enough insulin, or body doesn't use insulin correctly; therefore the individual needs to control their intake of carbohydrates. Some people can maintain normoglycaemia with diet alone, others need oral hypoglycaemic drugs and some may require insulin eventually
Usual age of onset	Less than 20 years	40–60 years
Control by oral hypoglycaemics	No	Yes; certainly in the first instance
Control by insulin	Yes	Not at the beginning of treatment but may be required as the disease progresses or if the patient remains unresponsive to therapy
Symptoms	Symptoms appear rapidly: frequent micturition; extreme hunger; extreme thirst; extreme weight loss; weakness and tiredness; feeling edgy and mood changes; nausea; vomiting; blurred vision	Symptoms appear slowly (the person may not feel any symptoms at all): increased thirst; increased micturition; feeling tired; feeling edgy; nausea; loss of weight; slow wound healing; recurrent infections of the skin, gums, vagina/penis and bladder; blurred vision; tingling or loss of sensation in hands or feet
Complications	Diabetic coma or ketoacidosis from hyperglycaemia; hypoglycaemia; nephropathy; blindness; myocardial infarction; cerebrovascular accident; peripheral vascular disease; neuropathy	Diabetic coma from hyperglycaemia; hypoglycaemia; nephropathy; blindness; myocardial infarction; cerebrovascular accident; peripheral vascular disease; neuropathy
Treatment	Carbohydrate controlled healthy diet; exercise; daily insulin; regular monitoring of blood glucose levels; monitoring of urine	Carbohydrate controlled healthy diet; exercise; regular monitoring of blood glucose levels; monitoring of urine

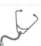

insulin). However, today it is almost entirely human. This is possible through a process called *recombinant DNA technology*, which involves inserting the DNA code for human insulin production into bacteria so that they then produce commercial amounts of insulin.

Insulin is destroyed in the GI system which is why you never see it given by mouth as a tablet, for example.

Once absorbed, insulin has a short half life of approximately 10 minutes. Therefore, for longer-term control, long-acting insulin is required (see p. 126).

Clinical tip

Insulin is usually given by injection. The commonest method of administration is by the SC route. It can be auto-injected by means of a device called a 'pen', although some patients prefer to use a small insulin pump. The newest device on the market at the moment is the insulin jet system which can be used on the abdomen, thighs or buttocks. It forces a very small stream of insulin through a nozzle placed on the skin. The jet of insulin is propelled with such force that it penetrates the skin without the need for a needle.

Short-acting insulins

Soluble insulin produces a quick and short-lived effect. It works in the same way as natural insulin by binding to the receptors on the cells and allowing glucose to enter. It also causes the cells in the liver, muscles and fat to increase their uptake of glucose from the blood. *Insulin lispro* is a special form of human insulin which works more rapidly but for a shorter period of time. This enables people to inject themselves just prior to eating a meal if they so wish.

These types of insulins are the only ones suitable for IV injection.

Clinical tip

An example of soluble insulin is *Actrapid*. When given subcutaneously it works within 30 to 60 minutes and its effects last for about eight hours. It is usually injected 15 to 30 minutes before a meal so that the increasing blood glucose levels after eating can be controlled. You will see these sorts of insulins being used in clinical practice as treatment for ketoacidosis where the regime is also called a 'sliding scale'. This means the insulin dose is determined by the person's blood glucose value, which is obtained at predetermined times (e.g. every two hours).

Intermediate insulins

Longer-acting preparations of insulin are made possible by mixing the insulin with a substance which slows its use in the body. An example of this is *isophane insulin* which starts working about an hour and a half after administration. Its maximum effect occurs between four and eight hours after administration and ends as long as 24 hours afterwards.

Clinical tip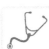

Isophane insulin is naturally white and cloudy in appearance and should not be used if it is not uniformly this colour after mixing. To mix the vial, gently roll it in your hands at least 10 times before administration.

Mixtard insulin contains a mixture of two types of insulin, soluble and isophane. Mixtard is available in a range of preparations containing these two insulins in differing proportions. Together, the combination is called *biphasic isophane insulin*. Pre-mixed combinations provide a rapid initial lowering of blood glucose, followed by a more prolonged effect that lasts throughout the day. This is thought to mimic the body's own insulin production more closely.

Long-acting insulins

By mixing insulin with protamine and zinc an even longer action can be elicited. *Lente* and *ultralente insulins* start working after 6 hours and last for 24 hours. *Insulin glargine* is modified insulin and is opposite in its effect to insulin lispro in that it is designed to provide a constant insulin supply and mimic even more closely the body's own physiological production of insulin. It is hoped that in conjunction with short-acting insulin a more normoglycaemic blood sugar can be maintained throughout a 24-hour period, lessening the risk of having a low blood sugar (hypoglycaemia) during the night. The National Institute for Health and Clinical Excellence (NICE) has endorsed the use of this insulin product in both type I and type II diabetes.

Side-effects

The main problem of giving insulin is that the blood sugar may be lowered too much, a state we call hypoglycaemia, which can cause brain damage. A person using insulin is three times more likely to be at risk from the effects of hypoglycaemia than a non-user.

Clinical tip

Patients suffering hypoglycaemia become dizzy, feel faint, begin to sweat and often appear to be drunk. The obvious way to treat this is to give sugar in the form of sweet drinks, glucose tablets or sugary snacks. If the person is unconscious, and this can occur relatively quickly, they will need IV glucose or intramuscular glucagon. Glucagon is a hormone which works in an opposite way to insulin and raises the blood glucose level by promoting the breakdown of stored glucose in the liver and muscles.

Insulin pumps

An insulin pump is portable and attached to the patient. It consists of a main pump unit which holds an insulin reservoir (usually 3ml capacity like the cartridges used in an insulin pen). The reservoir

---

Box 7.3 Types of insulin

Rapid acting analogue (clear)
Onset: 10–15 minutes
Peak: 60–90 minutes
Duration: 4–5 hours

Fast acting (clear)
Onset: 0.5–1 hour
Peak: 2–4 hours
Duration: 5–8 hours

Intermediate acting (cloudy)
Onset: 1–3 hours
Peak: 5–8 hours
Duration: Up to 18 hours

Long acting (cloudy)
Onset: 3–4 hours
Peak: 8–15 hours
Duration: 22–26 hours

Extended long acting analogue
Onset: 90 minutes
Duration: 24 hours

Premixed (cloudy)
Presented as a single vial which contains a fixed ratio (a percentage of rapid/fast acting to a percentage of intermediate/long acting)

---

is attached to a long, thin piece of tubing with a needle or cannula at one end which is known as the 'infusion set'.

To use the pump, the cartridge is filled with fast-acting insulin and fitted inside. There is no need to take long-acting insulin because the insulin pump delivers constant amounts to the body. The needle or cannula is inserted under the skin and held in place with an adhesive patch, which fixes to the surrounding skin. The other end of the tube is connected to the pump which then delivers insulin through the infusion set according to its programming.

Using a pump, patients can instantly change the insulin dose, and fast-acting insulin is more easily absorbed by the body. Because the body gets a constant, regular flow of insulin, the effect is more constant also.

Two types of dose are taken, basal and bolus. Modern insulin pumps allow users to regulate both doses at the same time and adjust the basal rate at any point. The basal rate is the same as a long-acting insulin regime for those diabetics without an insulin pump. This programme is consistent and regular, and controls the level of insulin into the bloodstream.

The bolus dose is designed to counteract the food being eaten. Therefore, when a diabetic eats a snack or at mealtimes the insulin pump can be programmed to provide an extra boost of insulin. Pumps can also be programmed to release a bolus dose over a longer period, which is be ideal for meals in restaurants and other similar occasions.

Oral hypoglycaemic agents

These are drugs that are usually given for type II diabetes. Dietary control certainly works for some people, however many others have difficulty in changing their lifestyles, especially on a permanent basis. For those people whose blood sugar is not controlled by diet alone there are a range of medicines available.

Metformin

Metformin is an antidiabetic medicine from a drug group called biguanides. It works in people with type II diabetes in three ways. First, it reduces the amount of glucose produced by cells in the liver. Second, it increases the sensitivity of muscle cells to insulin. Third, it delays movement of glucose from the GI tract to the blood following a meal. The cumulative effect of these processes is to lower the person's blood glucose level.

Metformin is described as being a first-line medicine in the treatment of type II diabetes. It can be used in combination with other antidiabetic medicines to provide better normoglycaemia.

The drug has a half life of approximately three hours and a dose of 500mg three times a day with or after food is usually prescribed. The most common side-effects are anorexia (lack of appetite), diarrhoea and nausea. An increase in lactic acid in the blood is a rare but potentially fatal consequence of taking the medication. This is more common in patients who already have kidney, liver or heart failure who should not be prescribed the drug.

Sulfonylureas

This classification of drug is also used in the treatment of type II diabetes, particularly in people whose diabetes cannot be controlled by diet alone. They work by stimulating the beta cells in the pancreas to secrete insulin. There are two generations of this type of medicine, first generation drugs such as tolbutamide and second generation drugs such as glipizide.

Tolbutamide comes as a tablet and is usually taken twice or three times a day. The drug may lead to hypoglycaemia, but, of the first generation drugs, it is probably the safest, especially with the elderly. Its duration of action is approximately six hours and therefore is less likely to cause hypoclycaemia.

Glipizide is a more potent drug than tolbutamide, however both are equally effective in their overall hypoglycaemic ability. This drug is usually well tolerated by patients, but hypoglycaemia is a usual side-effect.

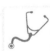

Clinical tip

Patients should be alerted to report symptoms such as shakiness, dizziness, sweating, sudden changes in behaviour and mood, and weakness as these may indicate a low blood sugar.

Oral hypoglycaemic agents such as tolbutamide and glipizide have been associated with increased cardiovascular mortality. However, there is no conclusive evidence that suggests that taking these drugs increases the risk of death from myocardial infarction.

There are some significant drug interactions with sulfonylureas, and certain drugs potentiate the hypoglycaemic effects. NSAIDs will lead to hypoglycaemia when given with sulfonureas. However, drugs such as thiazide diuretics and corticosteroids lessen the hypoglycaemic effects. This means that patients should have their blood glucose monitored more closely to ensure adequate control is maintained.

Meglitinides

Some drugs such as meglitnides that are not based on sulfonylureas have also been developed to expand the range of therapy. One such drug is nateglinide, which works in a similar way to sulfonylureas in that it enhances secretion of insulin from the beta cells in the pancreas. It is not as potent as most of the sulfonureas, is rapidly absorbed and has a fairly short elimination half life of three hours. This means that it has a short duration of action and there is therefore a lower risk of hypoglycaemia as a side-effect.

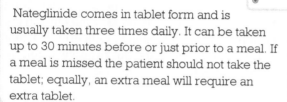

Clinical tip

Nateglinide comes in tablet form and is usually taken three times daily. It can be taken up to 30 minutes before or just prior to a meal. If a meal is missed the patient should not take the tablet; equally, an extra meal will require an extra tablet.

Thiazolidinediones (glitazones)

This class of drug came from a chance finding when it was being used as a fat-lowering treatment and it was noticed that thiazolidinediones also lowered blood glucose. The action of this class of drugs is complex. They reduce the breakdown of stored glucose in the liver and increase the amount of glucose entering muscle tissue. Insulin that is circulating is enhanced by these drugs. The accumulation of these actions leads to a lowering of the blood glucose level. They do not cause hypoglycaemia as a side-effect when used on their own but may do so if combined with insulin or a sulfonurea.

It is believed that this class of drugs also lowers fats that are thought to be implicated in the build up of fatty plaques in blood vessels (atherosclerosis). The only tablet in this group is pioglitazone. Its cardiovascular safety profile compares favorably with rosiglitazone (Avandia), which was with-

drawn after concerns about an increased risk of cardiac events. Pioglitazone is used on its own or alongside metformin and/or another antidiabetic medicine to treat type II (non-insulin dependent) diabetes mellitus. It can also be used with insulin. Pioglitazone comes as a tablet to take by mouth. It is usually taken once daily with or without meals. It should be taken at around the same time every day.

Clinical tip

You should inform the patient that it may take two weeks for their blood sugar to decrease and several weeks longer for them to feel the full effect of pioglitazone.

Common side-effects include nausea, difficulty in focusing, ankle swelling, increase in appetite and weight gain. Pioglitazone and other similar medications for diabetes may cause or worsen congestive heart failure (a condition in which the heart is unable to pump enough blood to the other parts of the body).

Alpha-glucosidase inhibitors

A drug called acarbose is used from this family of medicines to treat type II diabetes. It works by slowing down the action of chemicals in the body that break down foods which release glucose. Slowing food digestion helps to keep the blood glucose from rising very high after a meal.

The medicine is given as a tablet, usually three times a day. It is important that the patient takes each dose with the first bite of their meal. Side-effects include flatulence, diarrhoea, abdominal pain and bloating due to the amount of unabsorbed carbohydrates left in the GI system. Acarbose is not a treatment for diabetes that you will encounter often in a hospital setting although it is an option for patients.

Hypertension

Hypertension (high blood pressure) is associated with a risk of coronary heart disease. Increased

Box 7.4 Tablets used in type II diabetes

Drug group	Product name	Information
Biguanides	Metformin	Helps the cells of the body to use insulin. Does not cause hypoglycaemia as it does not stimulate the pancreas to secrete insulin. Does not cause weight gain. May cause nausea and vomiting
Sulfonylureas	Glipizide	Stimulates the pancreas to produce more insulin. Can cause hypoglycaemia. Can also lead to weight gain and therefore should be prescribed to people of normal weight
Meglitinides	Nateglinide (Starlix)	Increases the amount of insulin produced during a meal. Can be used alongside metformin
Thiazolidinediones	Rosiglitazone	Helps insulin sensitivity. May be used with either a sulphonurea or biguanide but not both. At present cannot be used alongside insulin
Alpha-glucosidase inhibitors	Acarbose (Glucobay)	Delays the rate at which sugars are digested. Side-effects include flatulence, a bloated feeling and diarrhoea. Can be used alongside other hypoglycaemic agents in this table

pressure in the blood vessels has a direct effect on the heart and vasculature. One of the major problems of having hypertension is that it has few symptoms and individuals often only discover they have the condition on routine screening. The effects of raised blood pressure have a pronounced effect on the heart, particularly the left ventricle. This increases in size (ventricular hypertrophy) as it attempts to pump against an increased peripheral resistance.

The arteries also respond to the increased pressure within them by enlargement of their muscular walls. This hypertrophy both in the heart and vessels leads to cardiac failure as a muscle cannot restore its normal contractility.

The risk of cerebral vascular accident (stroke) also rises significantly with elevation in systolic and diastolic pressures. Hypertensive disease is also associated with the formation of fatty plaques in the walls of blood vessels, a condition we call atherosclerosis. This is a Catch 22 situation as atherosclerosis leads to further hypertension. The combination of high pressure and artherosclerosis leads to weakness in the walls of arteries and increases the risk of them rupturing. The blood vessels most commonly affected are the cerebral, coronary and renal vessels. Therefore, as well as the increased risk of cerebral vascular accident and myocardial infarction, the individual is also likely to suffer from renal disease.

Hypertension may be defined as primary or secondary. In secondary hypertension the elevated blood pressure is caused by renal or endocrine disease. However, the majority of cases of hypertension are primary or 'essential' and this condition is still not fully understood. The causation of hypertension is most likely to be due to a number of interrelated factors which may be genetic or environmental.

Regardless of cause, hypertension is a fatal, silent killer, unless treated. In most instances the disease process extends over a long period of time and this is known as *benign hypertension*. However, in a small minority of cases the disease progresses very rapidly and is very difficult to control. This is referred to as *malignant hypertension* and is usually triggered by kidney disease arising from essential hypertension or other causes.

Arterial pressure is regulated by the performance of the heart (measured as cardiac output) and the diameter of the arterioles (total peripheral resistance). Hypertension involves an increase in either cardiac output or the peripheral resistance. Mechanisms that seem to be involved affect the extracellular fluid volume and expand the circulating blood volume. This involves excessive renin secretion from the kidney. Renin is a hormone that raises blood pressure in the body. Increased sympathetic activity which activates stress hormones and an excessive dietary salt intake, possibly associated with a low potassium intake, are also implicated in the pathogenesis of this disease.

Non-pharmacological remedies for hypertension are usually the first to be prescribed before commencing medicines. Weight reduction, salt restriction, moderation in alcohol consumption and cessation of smoking are all recommended before prescribing treatment. A GP may also prescribe a regime of moderate exercise which has been shown to be beneficial in helping to lower systolic pressure. Relaxation and biofeedback are also techniques that are advisable prior to drug therapy. It is important that the disease is diagnosed and treated early as intervention, be it pharmacological or non-pharmacological, can reduce the risk of much cardiovascular disease associated with hypertension.

In the past, treatment of hypertension involved giving patients medicines that had many side-effects, however, as medicine has progressed so has the pharmacology. Generally, patients are commenced on a thiazide diuretic. If this does not give adequate control then the patient may be prescribed drugs from the beta-adrenoreceptor antagonist (beta blocker) group. If the blood pressure remains elevated then the individual would progress onto more potent groups of drugs such as angiotensin-converting enzyme inhibitors, or calcium antagonists (calcium channel blockers). Finally a blockade of alpha adrenoreceptors would be commenced. Typically, drug regimes for peo-

ple with hypertension consist of a number of these drugs used in combination.

Thiazide diuretics

These are usually the first-line treatment for mild to moderate hypertension, providing there are no contraindications. A drug that is used commonly is bendroflumethiazide. You may come across other diuretic drugs such as frusimide. This works on a different part of the kidney (loop of henle). It is a more powerful diuretic and is not usually used for the treatment of hypertension.

Bendroflumethiazide works by stopping the body from selectively reabsorbing sodium. This has an effect on the circulating blood volume causing it to decrease. It has also been noted that this group of diuretics has an effect on blood vessels, causing them to vasodilate and lower blood pressure.

Bendroflumethiazide is well absorbed from the GI tract so is usually given as a tablet. A dose of 2.5mg daily is usually prescribed. Higher doses do not necessarily mean a greater fall in blood pressure, but would increase the side-effects. The maximum effect takes place at four to six hours and its duration of action is between 8 and 12 hours.

Problems can occur with this drug. First, it increases the amount of uric acid present in the plasma because it prevents that acid from being secreted from the body. Therefore, anybody suffering from gout should not take the medicine. Another common side-effect is potassium depletion.

Clinical tip

If a patient is a diabetic, controlling their blood sugar will become more difficult when taking drugs for high blood pressure. Male impotence can be caused by thiazide diuretics in about 20 per cent of individuals. However, this is reversible by stopping the medication. Caution should also be taken if the patient is receiving lithium for bipolar disorder as the diuretic can cause blood levels of lithium to become elevated.

Even on a small dose of 2.5mg of bendro-flumethiazide, the doctor should be carrying out routine urea and electrolyte blood investigations yearly. More significant side-effects can occur and the drug can cause hyperglycaemia.

Beta-adrenoreceptor antagonists

In practice these drugs are usually referred to as *beta blockers*. If a patient develops hypertension then taking this group of medicines will cause a gradual fall in arterial pressure. However, this will take several days or weeks to occur. How these drugs work is not fully understood but they appear to have actions that reduce the cardiac output, reduce renin production from the kidney and reduce the release of stress-related hormones such as adrenaline.

In the body you have at least two types of beta-adrenoreceptors, some in the heart (beta$_1$ receptors) and some in the lungs (beta$_2$ receptors). Beta blockers are either selective, whereby they stop the effect of adrenaline at beta$_1$ receptors, or non-selective whereby the drug blocks both types. This is a consideration as beta$_2$ receptors bring about bronchodilation. Therefore, blocking this effect in patients with airway disease is not desirable. Such patients should be given a selective drug such as atenolol.

This group of medicines can all be given in tablet form. Some are taken once daily (e.g. atenolol) and others need to be taken more often (e.g. propranolol). Serious side-effects are not common but are important when giving information to patients.

Patients with diabetes need to be informed that they might not recognize when they are going hypoglycaemic. The signs and symptoms of hypoglycaemia are mediated through the sympathetic nervous system. This group of drugs inhibits sympathetic responses and the patient may therefore get little warning of impending lowering of blood glucose levels.

Due to the fall in circulating blood volume, peripheral perfusion of tissues is a consideration. Often a person will complain of having cold hands and feet. Therefore, patients with peripheral vascular disease pose a particular problem and this type of medicine should be avoided. Other side-effects may include fatigue, a low pulse rate (bradycardia) and very vivid dreams and nightmares.

> **Clinical tip**
>
> One way you can usually identify a drug from this group is that it ends in 'olol' (e.g. atenolol).

Angiotensin-converting enzyme inhibitors

These are known as *ACE inhibitors* and work by stopping the powerful vasoconstricting effects of angiotensin II on the blood vessels. In order to become active angiotensin II has to convert from angiotensin I. This group of drugs, which includes captopril, stops this conversion from taking place, therefore lowering the blood pressure.

It is important that the patient drinks plenty of fluids while on these drugs. Dehydration lowers the blood pressure further, so causing an unwanted severe hypotensive state. Captopril can be used on its own or in combination with other antihypertensive agents. It is a powerful hypotensive drug and therefore patients usually start on a low dose.

Sometimes it is advisable to take the initial dose of the drug before going to bed, so removing the chances of faints or falls due to hypotension.

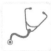

> **Clinical tip**
>
> Most drugs ending in 'pril' are usually from the ACE inhibitor group (e.g. captopril).

A dry cough from irritation of the bronchial mucosa is a common side-effect with some patients going on to experience bronchospasm. Captopril has certain individual side-effects due to the nature of its biochemistry. It can cause rashes, changes in taste, a lowering of a group of white cells called neutrophils (neutropenia) and protein to appear in the urine (proteinurea).

Other drugs in this group such as lisinopril and ramipril will not cause the same degree of side-effects as captopril because their chemical structure is slightly different. Patients who have a narrowing of their renal artery (renal artery stenosis) will develop renal failure if treated with this group of drugs as their bodies depend on a fully functioning renin angiotensin cycle.

Calcium antagonists

These drugs act by limiting the amount of calcium that enters smooth and cardiac muscle. This causes the blood vessels to dilate, therefore causing the blood pressure to fall. Some of these drugs act better on the heart muscle (e.g. verapamil) and others work better on smooth muscle of the blood vessels (e.g. nifedipine and amlodipine).

Calcium antagonists are well absorbed by the GI system and are given in tablet form. However, drugs differ in how short- or long-acting they are and this has an effect on dosage and unwanted side-effects. For example, nifedipine has a short half life and needs to be taken more frequently than amlodipine which is taken once a day. However, slow release preparations of nifedipine are available.

Unwanted side-effects are an extension of the drug's therapeutic activities. Shorter-acting medicines may cause flushing and headaches and if used over a long period of time can cause ankle swelling. Apart from these predictable side-effects these drugs are relatively trouble-free.

Alpha-adrenoreceptor antagonists

A drug called prazosin was the first selective alpha antagonist to be developed and was used for many years. However, better drugs have now been developed, for example doxazosin and terazosin. These can be taken once a day.

Like beta blockers, these drugs work by inhibiting the action of adrenaline and noradrenaline on body systems. The drugs mentioned above are highly selective, which means they can affect vessels, so causing dilatation, but do not speed up the heart rate (tachycardia). Neither do they lead to any appreciable severe lowering of blood pressure

when standing (postural hypotension). Perhaps for these reasons that they have become more popular, especially in combination with other antihypertensive therapies.

Parkinson's disease

This is a progressive disorder of movement. Certain neurones in part of the brain called the *basal nuclei* degenerate and this leads to a lack of a neurotransmitter called dopamine. Typically, this disease occurs in people who are over the age of 50. The reduction in the release of dopamine causes the basal nuclei to become overactive and this overactivity presents itself in a number of ways. The patient develops a persistent tremor, even at rest, and quite often there are head-nodding and pill-rolling movements of the fingers. Their posture becomes affected and they begin to bend forward and walk in small, shuffling steps. Textbooks used to describe the person's face as 'mask-like' because they acquire a stiff facial expression. Finally, the patient has trouble in initiating and coordinating movement.

Parkinson's disease was first described by James Parkinson in 1817. In 1960 Hornykiewicz demonstrated that the dopamine content of the substantia nigra in post-mortem examination of patients with the disease was extremely low – in some cases 10 per cent less than normal. More sophisticated diagnostic tests have revealed similar findings and suggest the loss of dopamine occurs over several years. Symptoms only show themselves when the dopamine content of this area has fallen below between 20 and 40 per cent of the normal.

With this knowledge, one would expect to be able to find a cure. It would seem on the face of it that all we need to do is replace the lost dopamine and the patient would return to a normal state. Drugs that are given for this debilitating disease do work by increasing dopamine in the brain in a number of ways, however despite these pharmacological interventions patients do *not* return to a normal state. Many deteriorate and suffer dementia. In addition to the affects of the disease there are also side-effects to the medication.

Box 7.5 Drugs used in hypertension

Younger than 55	
Step 1	Angiotensin-converting enzyme inhibitor (ACE inhibitor)
Step 2	ACE inhibitor **PLUS** Calcium channel blocker or thiazide-type diuretic
Step 3	ACE inhibitor **PLUS** Calcium channel blocker **PLUS** Thiazide-type diuretic
Step 4	ACE inhibitor **PLUS** Calcium channel blocker **PLUS** Thiazide-type diuretic **PLUS** Further diuretic or alpha blocker or beta blocker
Older than 55 or black patients of any age	
Step 1	Calcium channel blocker or thiazide-type diuretic
Step 2	ACE inhibitor **PLUS** Calcium channel blocker or thiazide-type diuretic
Step 3	ACE inhibitor **PLUS** Calcium channel blocker **PLUS** Thiazide-type diuretic
Step 4	ACE inhibitor **PLUS** Calcium channel blocker **PLUS** Thiazide-type diuretic **PLUS** Further diuretic or alpha blocker or beta blocker
Taken from the NICE clinical guideline 34 (2006)	

Levodopa

This remains the first line treatment for Parkinson's disease. You cannot give pure dopamine as the BBB will not allow it to enter and it is also de-stroyed quickly by enzymes in the peripheral tissues. Levodopa is a drug that can cross the BBB and then be converted by the central nervous system into dopamine. It is nearly always combined with another substance that stops peripheral enzymes breaking down dopamine. This means that generally more levodopa is available to the brain and also a lower dose of dopamine can be given as most of it remains intact rather than being destroyed by enzymes. Examples of medicines that are combined or given with levodopa are carbidopa and benserazide.

When given levodopa the response rates of patients are good. Some studies suggest that 20 per cent of patients may actually be restored to normal function for a while. However, this improvement is often only short-lived and as time goes by the levodopa becomes less effective. This loss of efficacy is probably due to the unrelenting course of the disease.

Two major side-effects are associated with giving levodopa. First, a condition called dyskinesia can develop which means that the individual develops a series of involuntary movements, causing acute embarrassment as they usually affect the face and limbs. If the dose is lowered, the dyskinesia does stop, but is replaced by the rigidity it had improved. This is a fine line that the patient and doctor walk in order to accept the consequences of both illness and treatment.

A second side-effect associated with this drug group is called the 'on-off ' effect. This is where, quite suddenly, the drug therapy seems to stop working. This can be quite distressing for the patient and can sometimes occur when they are in the middle of doing something. The reason for this fluctuation is not fully understood, however, patients should be made aware of both these side-effects when commencing treatment.

The patient may also suffer more short-term side-effects from the medication, though these quite often improve over a period of time. They may feel sick, have no appetite and suffer a slight drop in blood pressure. This decrease in blood pressure could have a more serious effect if the patient is having antihypertensive therapy as they could develop postural hypotension.

A small number of patients may develop delusions and hallucinations as the brain is given extra dopamine which is thought to mimic the high levels found in patients with schizophrenia.

Selegiline

This medicine works by stopping the enzyme that breaks down dopamine in the synapses, therefore making more dopamine available. The enzyme is called monoamine oxidase-B and appears only in regions of the brain which are dopamine rich. This means that the drug only works in these areas of the brain, so limiting any side-effects or interactions. Giving this drug with levodopa seems to have better results than giving levodopa on its own. However, when levodopa is given in combination with either carbidopa or benserazide, there is no difference noted between this and giving selegiline only.

Dopamine receptor agonists

This group of drugs works by mimicking the action of dopamine on dopamine receptors. Examples of this class are bromocriptine and pergolide. Their duration of action is longer than that of levodopa so they do not need to be given as often. The toxic effects of these drugs are similar to levodopa, however, the schizophrenic-type symptoms can be more severe. Sometimes these drugs are given in combination with levodopa in order to reduce overall side-effects or improve the patient's response.

Acetylcholine antagonists

Prior to the discovery of levodopa this group of drugs was the main treatment for patients suffering from Parkinson's disease. Dopamine works opposite to acetylcholine in the nigra striatel system, therefore if dopamine is lacking, by stopping the actions of acetylcholine, balance can be restored albeit at a lower level. This is the thinking behind acetylcholine antagonists. The action of drugs like benzatropine is more limited than levodopa in that they do not reduce rigidity significantly.

These drugs also have troublesome side-effects that can lead to glaucoma and urinary retention in an elderly person. As a result their use is usually confined to treating side-effects of drugs given as neuroleptic agents (e.g. chlorpromazine). However, with the advent of atypical antipsychotic

Box 7.6 Drugs used in Parkinson's disease

Drug type	Generic name	Information
Dopamine precursor. Added agents are peripheral dopamine decarboxylation inhibitors	Levodopa + benserazide/carbidopa/entacapone	Benserazide, carbidopa and entacapone irreversibly inhibit monamine oxidase type B to decrease metabolism of dopamine. Decrease in nausea. Used for idiopathic, postencephalitic and symptomatic Parkinson's disease especially in patients who are rigid, have bradykinesia or are elderly. Controlled release (CR) tablets may be useful to take at night if having 'off' periods the following morning. May slow progression or severity of symptoms
Inhibits monoamine oxidase B to decrease metabolism of dopamine	Selegiline	Add-on therapy for Parkinson's disease (may aid wearing-off effects). Improves disability scores, may decrease freezing. Mild symptomatic benefit
Dopamine agonists	Bromocriptine Cabergoline Pergolide Pramipexole Ropinirole	Idiopathic Parkinson's disease, restless leg syndrome. Dopamine agonists may have fewer motor complications but an increased risk of hallucinations, sleepiness or ankle oedema (excess fluid). May be preferable in younger patients. May help to reduce the dose of levodopa required for same effect
Anticholinergic agents (block cholinergic activity in the brain)	Benzotropine Esthopropazine Procyclidine Trihexyphenidyl	Tremor in Parkinson's disease, foot dystonia, excessive drooling, drug-induced extra-pyramidal symptoms, motor function

medication their use is in decline. Refer to Chapter 8 for more on drugs that are used in mental health.

Epilepsy

Epilepsy is the most common chronic disabling condition of the nervous system. Epileptic seizures result from an imbalance of the excitatory and inhibitory mechanisms within the brain, the nerve impulses generated from the neurones being abnormal and uncoordinated. The form of seizure that the person suffers usually depends on the part of the brain affected. Seizures can range from brief lapses in attention to full-blown convulsive fits which may last up to several minutes. The classification of epilepsy recognizes two major categories: *partial* and *generalized*.

Partial seizures

These tend to occur in a localized area of the brain. The symptoms depend on which brain region is discharging these abnormal impulses. Simple partial seizures are an example of this, where the motor cortex is irritated, resulting in twitching. The patient does not lose consciousness. The twitching sometimes spreads from a small area of the body to a larger area as the impulse spreads across the motor cortex. This is called a *Jacksonian seizure*.

Complex partial seizures usually originate from the temporal lobe and are preceded by what is called an *aura* or *warning*. The person then commences to enter into a period of altered behaviour where they repeat movements over and over again.

Examples of this may be rubbing, patting or plucking activities. Patients may also describe alterations in sensation like a smell or a sense of being there before (déjà vu). These seizures may last a few minutes, after which the person has no memory of the events. The behaviours during these seizures can be bizarre and accompanied by strong emotional responses, for example aggression.

Generalized seizures

These involve the whole brain and affect the reticular formation centres responsible for consciousness and arousal. Abnormal impulses arise throughout both hemispheres. Two important categories are *absent seizures* which used to be called *petit mal* and *tonic clonic seizures* which used to be called *grand mal*.

Absent seizures are characterized by a brief alteration in consciousness which is sometimes very difficult to see. This type of seizure happens more in children and can be frequent in nature.

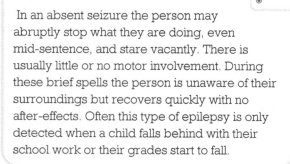

Clinical tip

In an absent seizure the person may abruptly stop what they are doing, even mid-sentence, and stare vacantly. There is usually little or no motor involvement. During these brief spells the person is unaware of their surroundings but recovers quickly with no after-effects. Often this type of epilepsy is only detected when a child falls behind with their school work or their grades start to fall.

Tonic clonic seizures are vastly different. These consist of an initial strong contraction of the whole muscular system causing a rigid spasm. Respira-

tion ceases with defecation, micturition and salivation often occurring. This tonic stage lasts for approximately a minute. The person then begins to suffer a series of violent rhythmic jerking movements of the limbs. They usually develop an increased heart rate (tachycardia) and begin to sweat. This phase lasts about two to four minutes, followed by a coma. The person is usually sleepy after the seizure and often cannot remember the event.

Clinical tip

A condition known as *status epilepticus* can occur in some patients, where one tonic clonic seizure follows another. This may continue for a period of time and can become life-threatening. Medical treatment needs to be implemented urgently in such cases.

Treatment for epilepsy is aimed at producing a life free of seizures. In order for this to be achieved patients are prescribed a range of drugs which are called *anticonvulsants*. These medicines work in one of three ways. Some block sodium channels in the neurone, others block calcium channels and the third group enhance an inhibitory neurotransmitter called gamma-aminobutyric acid (GABA).

Inhibition of sodium channel function

In Chapter 3 we discussed the firing of a neurone (see p. 32) and the importance of the passage of sodium into the neurone. It can be deduced that if we block this action in some way, then neurones will be less likely to fire. Sodium-inhibiting drugs do not block all sodium channels but are selective to channels that allow high frequency impulses to take place. In other words, they dampen down the excitability in neurones without switching them off. An example of this class of drug is phenytoin.

Phenytoin

This drug is still widely used but not for absent seizures, which may get worse if the drug is administered. It is well absorbed by the body when given orally but has certain characteristic pharmacokinetic tendencies which must be taken into consideration before it is prescribed. First, it binds to plasma proteins in the blood, which is not unusual for drugs to do, however when giving drugs that unblock this mechanism (e.g. salicylates) there is an increase of the phenytoin in the person's plasma. Phenytoin also increases enzymes into the liver that can affect the breakdown (metabolism) of other drugs that the patient may be taking. This process is called *enzyme induction*. For example, if the patient is taking oral anticoagulants the effect of these will be unpredictable if phenytoin is also given.

Phenytoin works to its full potential between 40 and 100 micromoles per litre. If the range exceeds this the patient gets more toxic side-effects without any further protection from seizures. This is why it is important to impress upon the patient the need for regular blood monitoring while on this therapy.

Side-effects begin to appear when the dose pushes the blood plasma levels to over 100 micromoles per litre and become severe if the blood plasma increased beyond 150 micromoles per litre. The patient may complain of feeling dizzy (vertigo), have headaches and their movements may become shaky. They may have difficulty walking (ataxia). In some cases people begin to have involuntary rapid movement of their eyes, a condition we call *nystagmus*. If the blood levels begin to rise further, the patient becomes confused and there is marked intellectual impairment. One particularly unpleasant side-effect of this drug is the development of swelling of the gums. This is called *hyperplasia* and can often be disfiguring and therefore acutely embarrassing.

Phenytoin has also been responsible for malformations in babies born to women taking the drug. Problems such as cleft palate were increased more than in the general population, therefore if a woman falls pregnant while taking the medication she should seek professional advice immediately.

Inhibition of calcium channels

Some of the anticonvulsant drugs are thought to have minor involvement in blocking calcium channels. Indeed, gabapentin, a fairly recent addition to the anticonvulsant range, may have some action on calcium channels. The only drug known for its action purely on calcium uptake in the neurone is ethosuximide.

Ethosuximide

This is the first line management drug when it comes to treatment for absent seizures. It has little or no effect in other types of epilepsy and can sometimes actually increase the risk of seizures.

The drug works on a certain class of calcium channels. It is thought that through their action they moderate the firing of neurones in an area of the brain called the *thalamus*. The abnormal firing of neurones in this area seems to play a role in the generation of absent seizures. The dose of the drug in adults is usually 0.5–2g daily. In children it falls to 10–20mg per kg once a day.

Side-effects are relatively minor but obviously troublesome if you are the one taking the medication. They include nausea, anorexia and sometimes lethargy and dizziness. Very rarely the drug can have severe hypersensitivity reactions.

Enhancement of GABA action

Sodium valproate

It is not entirely clear exactly how valproate works as it does several things in the brain. First, the chemical messenger (or neurotransmitter) GABA is 'inhibitory' on the brain – i.e. it calms the brain down. Once it has worked there are other chemicals (or enzymes) in the brain which are there to break GABA down so that it can no longer work. In people with normal levels of GABA this prevents there being too much GABA. In some people it is thought that there may not be enough GABA in the brain. This lack seems to 'trigger' fits or overactivity. Valproate helps to stop the breakdown of GABA and so leaves enough of this chemical in the brain to help prevent fits.

Second, it may inhibit 'repetitive firing' of neurones. When a message is passed, there is a short refractory period or gap (about one thousandth of a second) before the next message can be passed, during which time the nerve ending resets itself.

Valproate may increase this refractory period or time by a small amount. Under normal circumstances, this will make no difference at all, but if the brain is overactive and lots of messages are being passed in quick succession the valproate will reduce the number of messages back to the normal level (e.g. if the next message follows along before the nerve has reset itself, the message can't be passed).

Compared with other anticonvulsant drugs, valproate is relatively free of unwanted side-effects, however the patient should be informed that they may feel sleepy to start with and so need to take extra care when driving or operating any type of machinery. This effect should wear off after the patient has been taking the medicine for a while. Valproate can cause some people to become more hungry than usual and they may then put on weight. Some patients may put on weight even without eating more. The patient should be informed to see a dietician for advice if weight gain becomes problematic.

Clinical tip

Valproate can be given by a variety of routes. The starting dose is usually 600mg daily after food but this may be increased. It is especially important that the patient swallows enteric-coated tablets or capsules whole. These tablets should not be crushed or chewed. The coating helps to prevent stomach upsets. Crushing or chewing will cause the drug to be released too soon and may result in side-effects. Sodium valproate tablets which are not enteric coated (i.e. Epilim 100mg) may be crushed if necessary.

The most serious side-effect is poisoning of the liver (hepatotoxicity). For the first six months of treatment the patient will need a regular blood test (e.g. every month) to check that the drug is not affecting their liver. The patient may also need to have blood tests from time to time to make sure that the dose of valproate is enough and not too much or too little for them.

It is also important for the patient to consider that there will be a risk from taking this medicine during pregnancy. Major malformations occur spontaneously in about 2–4 per cent of all pregnancies, even if no drugs are taken. A medicine causing teratogenicity (foetal malformation) is called a teratogen. Since a baby has completed its main development between days 17 and 60 of the pregnancy (the so-called 'first trimester'), these first 2 to 16 weeks are the main concern. After that, there may be other problems (e.g. some medicines may cause slower growth). The infant may also be affected after birth (e.g. withdrawal effects are possible with some drugs). There is some evidence of problems of this nature when taking valproate (e.g. a 1 in 100 chance of spina bifida and a 'valproate syndrome'). Therefore this drug is not normally given in pregnancy.

Vigabatrin

Vigabatrin works by stopping the breakdown of GABA in the brain by the enzyme GABA transaminase. The drug is extremely specific for this enzyme, so enhancing the inhibitory effects of GABA in humans. It is well absorbed from the GI tract and is therefore given as a tablet. It has a short plasma half life but because it blocks the GABA-destroying enzyme irreversibly it can be given once daily. The body will obviously make more GABA transaminase so the drug has to be given continuously. The main side-effects are depression and psychotic disturbances.

Clinical tip

Patients can become quite hostile and aggressive on receiving this medication. The drug is often tried on patients for whom conventional therapy has failed to reduce their seizures.

Box 7.7 Drugs used in the treatment of epilepsy

Drug	Use	Side-effects
First line anticonvulsant drugs		
Sodium valproate	Effective against generalized tonic clonic seizures, partial seizures and absences	Can cause drowsiness, tremors, reversible hair loss, weight gain. Can cause liver damage. Can make polycystic ovary syndrome worse. May cause menstrual irregularities. High risk of foetal abnormalities
Ethosuximide	Effective against absences only	Can cause nausea and drowsiness initially. May cause anorexia and weight loss
Second line anticonvulsant drugs		
Phenytoin	Effective against generalized tonic clonic seizures and partial seizures. Ineffective against absences	Blood tests essential to guide dosing. May cause skin rash, drowsiness, ataxia and slurred speech. Overgrowth of the gums, excess hair growth, acne and some anaemias may occur with prolonged treatment
Vigabatrin	Effective against partial seizures and secondarily generalized seizures where all previous treatment has been ineffective. May worsen myoclonic and absent seizures	May cause drowsiness, behavioural and mood changes. One in every three people currently taking this medication report visual field problems. Psychotic reactions have been reported

Case studies

① Joseph Olita, a 30-year-old man, has been on salbutamol inhaler and inhaled steroids for many years. His asthma has never really been under control and the requirement of steroid and beta-agonist usage has increased steadily. It is suspected that Joseph has not been using his inhalers properly. You are asked to reinforce this patient's technique. What steps would you take the patient through and what advice would you give? Discuss with reference to:

- The mode of action of the two medicines.
- The correct inhaler technique.
- The language you would use in teaching Joseph this technique.

② Elizabeth Jones is 11 years old and is asthmatic. Her asthma is well controlled on the following medication: a salbutamol 'easibreath' device, two puffs as required for breathlessness; an inhaled corticosteroid prophylaxis. Elizabeth is moving up to high school and is embarrassed about using her inhalers in front of her classmates. Explain to her the benefits of preventative use of her steroid inhaler and the necessity of using her salbutamol to prevent severe asthma attack. Discuss with reference to:

- Corticosteroid action on the airways and bronchodilation produced by salbutamol.
- Assuaging Elizabeth's concerns.

Key learning points

Introduction

➤ Chronic diseases are brought about by demographic, environmental and lifestyle changes.
➤ Common conditions include asthma, diabetes, hypertension, Parkinson's disease and epilepsy.

Asthma

➤ Can be described as acute and chronic.
➤ Triggered by chemicals, foreign proteins and cold air.
➤ Respiratory changes triggered by an allergic response.
➤ Histamine is released causing bronchoconstriction.
➤ Swelling and excess mucous production is present.

Asthma in children

➤ Affects as many as 15 per cent of children in the UK.
➤ There are many risk factors for developing childhood asthma.
➤ Diagnosis of asthma in children is difficult because of its complex nature.
➤ Most asthma medications can safely be prescribed for younger children.

Drugs used in treating asthma

➤ Two groups are used: bronchodilators and inhaled anti-inflammatories.
➤ Examples of bronchodilators are salbutamol and theophylline.
➤ Examples of inhaled corticosteroids are beclomethasone and budesonide.
➤ Candidiasis can be a problem with inhaled corticosteroids.
➤ Inhaler technique is an important part of patient education.
➤ Cromoglicate is given as a preventative drug.

Chronic obstructive pulmonary disease

➤ A general term which includes the conditions chronic bronchitis and emphysema.
➤ The most common cause is smoking.
➤ Difficulty with breathing may eventually become distressing.
➤ Drugs that may be considered beta-agonists, antimuscarinics and theophylline.

Diabetes

➤ A chronic metabolic disease.
➤ Two types: insulin dependent and non-insulin dependent.
➤ Complications of the disease produce macrovascular and microvascular problems.

→

Medicine management of diabetes

➢ Treatment aims at achieving normoglycaemia.
➢ Insulin is prepared in different lengths of action.
➢ Insulin is given by SC injection.
➢ Giving insulin can cause hypoglycaemia.
➢ Oral hypoglycaemics can be used in non-insulin dependent diabetes mellitus.
➢ Examples of oral hypoglycaemics are metformin, glipizede, nateglinide and pioglitazone.

Hypertension

➢ High blood pressure has pronounced effects on the heart.
➢ It is associated with atherosclerosis.
➢ Lifestyle changes are the first course of action in treatment.
➢ Main classes of drugs are thiazide, diuretics, beta-adrenoreceptor antagonists, angiotensin-converting enzyme inhibitors, calcium antagonists or blockers and alpha-adrenoreceptor antagonists.
➢ Drugs are often given in combination therapy.
➢ Patients usually start with thiazides and progress to more powerful agents.

Parkinson's disease

➢ Progressive disorder of movement due to lack of the neurotransmitter dopamine.
➢ Persistent tremor, head nodding and pill-rolling are examples of movement disorder.
➢ Drugs used in the treatment process include levodopa, selegiline and dopamine receptor agonists.
➢ Drugs do not offer a cure.

Epilepsy

➢ Common disabling neurological condition.
➢ Classified into partial seizures and generalized seizures.
➢ Drugs used inhibit sodium and calcium channels in the neuronal membrane and also increase the amount of GABA.
➢ Phenytoin is an anticonvulsant drug which is highly protein bound.
➢ Phenytoin can have unpleasant side-effects such as ataxia and vertigo.
➢ Ethosuximide is used only in absent seizures.
➢ Sodium valproate increases GABA.
➢ Need to check blood levels of patients taking anticonvulsants.
➢ Vigabatrin is a new drug which raises the level of GABA.

Calculations

1 A patient requires intramuscular furosimide 20mg. Your stock ampoule contains 40mg in 4ml. How many ml would you draw up?

2 Sodium valproate suspension 200mg is prescribed for an individual. You only have 125mg in 5ml. How many ml would you give?

3 Bendroflumethiazide 7.5mg is prescribed orally. Your stock tablets are 2.5mg. How many tablets would you give?

4 Your mentor asks you to check a dose of medication for IV injection. The patient requires amino-phylline 50mg and the ampoule comes as 250mg in 10ml. How much should have been drawn into the syringe?

5 Sodium valproate suspension 50mg is prescribed for an individual. You only have 200mg in 5ml. How many ml would you give?

6 A child requires 50mg of phenobarbitone. If the stock ampoules contain 200mg in 2ml, how much will you draw up?

7 A patient requires 1mg of bumetanide, you have a stock ampoule containing 2mg in 4ml. How much do you give?

8 Carbamazipine 0.25g is needed; your suspension contains 100mg in 5ml. How much would you administer?

9 You have a vial of actrapid containing 100 units per ml. How much do you need to give 28 units?

10 Sodium valproate suspension 90mg is approximately equivalent to 100mg capsules or tablets. You have a patient with swallowing difficulties. How many ml of suspension (30mg in 5ml) should you give for a dose of 300mg capsules?

For further assistance with calculations, please see Meriel Hutton's *Essential Calculation Skills for Nurses, Midwives and Healthcare Practitioners* (Open University Press 2009).

Multiple choice questions

Try answering these multiple choice questions to test what you have learned from reading this chapter. You can check your answers on page 201.

1 Which of the following drugs is a beta 2 agonist used in the treatment of asthma?

a) Ipratropium
b) Salbutamol
c) Beclometasone
d) Theophylline

←

2 What measures might be employed to help reduce the possibility of developing oral candidiasis when using inhaled corticosteroids?

a) Using a spacer and altering the inhaler technique
b) Altering the inhaler technique and taking antifungal lozenges
c) Rinsing the mouth and altering their inhaler technique
d) Using a spacer and rinsing the mouth after taking the medication

3 Glipizide belongs to which family of hypoglycaemics?

a) Sulfonylureas
b) Biguanides
c) Meglitinides
d) Glitazones

4 Insulin is given by injection because

a) It is cheaper to give it that way
b) It takes a long time to absorb it from the GI tract
c) It is destroyed in the GI tract
d) A tablet has not yet been developed

5 Which of the following drugs is a calcium channel blocker?

a) Bendroflumethiazide
b) Captopril
c) Nifedipine
d) Prazosin

6 Which drug group would be the first line management of mild to moderate hypertension?

a) Beta-adrenoreceptor antagonists
b) Diuretics
c) Calcium antagonists
d) Alpha-adrenoreceptor antagonists

7 Levodopa is often given with which other drug in treating Parkinson's disease?

a) Pergolide
b) Benzatropine
c) Selegiline
d) Carbidopa

←

8 Parkinson's disease is caused by a lack of which substance?

a) Acetylcholine
b) Dopamine
c) Serotonin
d) Noradrenaline

9 The drug of choice in treating absences is

a) Ethosuximide
b) Gabapentin
c) Phenytoin
d) Sodium valproate

10 Which of the following neurotransmitters has an inhibitory function?

a) Noradrenaline
b) Acetylcholine
c) Gamma amino butyric acid
d) Serotonin

Recommended further reading

Beckwith, S. and Franklin, P. (2007) *Oxford Handbook of Nurse Prescribing*. Oxford: Oxford University Press.

Bourke, S.J. (2007) *Respiratory Medicine*, 7th edn. Malden, MA: Blackwell.

Brenner, G.M. and Stevens, C.W. (2006) *Pharmacology*, 2nd edn. Philadelphia, PA: Saunders Elsevier.

Campbell, D.A. (2006) Respiratory nursing: understanding difficult-to-control asthma, *Nursing Times*, 102(36): 44–5.

Capaldi, B. (2005) Treatments and devices for future diabetes management, *Nursing Times*, 101(18): 30–2.

Clark, A. (2002) Spotlight: drug information factsheet – diuretics, *Professional Nurse*, 17(8): 484.

Clayton, B.D. (2009) *Basic Pharmacology for Nurses*, 15th edn. St. Louis, MO: Mosby Elsevier.

Coben, D. and Atere-Roberts, E. (2005) *Calculations for Nursing and Healthcare*, 2nd edn. Basingstoke: Palgrave Macmillan.

Cradock, S. (2004) Essential reading on type 1 diabetes, *Nursing Standard*, 18(49): 29.

Cradock, S. and Skinner, C. (2001) Managing type 2 diabetes: a dynamic approach, *Nursing Times*, 97(7): 42–3.

Doran, C. (2000) Learning curve: managing epilepsy, *Nursing Times*, 96(19): 37–8.

Downie, G., Mackenzie, J. and Williams, A. (2007) *Pharmacology and Medicines Management for Nurses*, 4th edn. Edinburgh: Churchill Livingstone.

Durham, S.R. (2008) *ABC of Allergies*. Malden, MA: Blackwell.

Everett, J. (2004) The role of insulin pumps in the management of diabetes, *Nursing Times*, 100(16): 48–9.

Gallimore, D. and Jordan, S. (2004) Prescription drugs, uses and effects: ACE inhibitors – cardiovascular disease, *Nursing Standard*, 18(45).

Gatford, J.D. and Phillips, N. (2006) *Nursing Calculations*, 7th edn. Edinburgh: Churchill Livingstone Elsevier.

Hainsworth, T. (2005) NT clinical: how to maintain optimal glycaemic control in diabetes, *Nursing Times*, 101(48): 19–20.

Hewitt, J. and Jordan, S. (2005) Antiepileptics: neurology, *Nursing Standard*, 19(49).

Hill, J. (2003) Diabetes: devices for insulin administration, *Nursing Times*, 99(15): 51–2.

Hill, J. (2005) The use of insulin to improve treatment in type 2 diabetes, *Nursing Times*, 101(28): 32–4.

Hillson, R. (2002) *Practical Diabetes Care*, 2nd edn. Oxford: Oxford University Press.

Jarvis, J., Burden, A. and Burden, M.L. (2004) An RCT into calculating insulin start dose in type 2 diabetes, *Nursing Times*, 100(21): 40–4.

Jordan, S. and Griffiths, H. (2004) Prescription drugs, uses and effects: diuretics – cardiovascular disease, *Nursing Standard*, 18(37).

Jordan, S. and Lake, R. (2005) Insulin, *Nursing Standard*, 19(32).

Karch, A.M. (2008) *Focus on Nursing Pharmacology*, 4th edn. Philadelphia, PA: Lippincott Williams & Wilkins.

Lapham, R. and Agar, H. (2003) *Drug Calculations for Nurses: A Step-by-step Approach*, 2nd edn. London: Arnold.

Levy, D. (2006) *Practical Diabetes*, 2nd edn. St. Albans: Altman Publishing.

Lowey, A. (2005) Drug treatment of type 2 diabetes in adults, *Nursing Standard*, 20(11): 55–64, 66, 68.

McLoughlin, C. (2004) Diuretic drugs, *Professional Nurse*, 20(2): 50–1.

Nair, M. (2007) Diabetes management: nursing management of the person with diabetes mellitus – part 2, *British Journal of Nursing*, 16(4): 232–5.

Newell, K. and Hume, S. (2006) Choosing the right inhaler for patients with asthma, *Nursing Standard*, 21: 46–8.

NICE (National Institute for Clinical Excellence) (2002) *Clinical Guideline G: Type 2 Diabetes, Blood Glucose*. London: NICE.

NICE (National Institute for Clinical Excellence) (2002) *Clinical Guideline H: Type 2 Diabetes, Management of Blood Pressure and Blood Lipids*. London: NICE.

NICE (National Institute for Clinical Excellence) (2003) NICE approval for epilepsy drugs, *Nursing Times*, 99(46): 6.

NICE (National Institute for Clinical Excellence) (2004) *Clinical Guideline 5: Chronic Obstructive Pulmonary Disease*. London: NICE.

NICE (National Institute for Clinical Excellence) (2004) *Clinical Guideline 15: Type 1 Diabetes*. London: NICE.

NICE (National Institute for Clinical Excellence) (2004) *Clinical Guideline 20: Epilepsy*. London: NICE.

NICE (National Institute for Health and Clinical Excellence) (2006) *Clinical Guideline 34: Hypertension*. London: NICE.

NICE (National Institute for Health and Clinical Excellence) (2006) *Clinical Guideline 35: Parkinson's Disease*. London: NICE.

Noble, C. (2006) Modes of drug delivery used to manage Parkinson's disease, *Nursing Times*, 102(32): 30–2.

Nursing Times (2003) What you need to know about … asthma, *Nursing Times*, 99(18): 28.

Nursing Times (2004) What you need to know about … insulin. *Nursing Times*, 100(8): 29.

O'Connor, B. (2001) Inhaler devices: compliance with steroid therapy, *Nursing Standard*, 15(48): 40–2.

Phillips, A. (2007) Experiences of patients with type 2 diabetes starting insulin therapy, *Nursing Standard*, 21(23): 35–41.

Phillips, A. (2007) Starting patients on insulin therapy: diabetes nurse specialist views, *Nursing Standard*, 21(30): 35–40.

Rees, J. and Kanabar, D. (2006) *ABC of Asthma*, 5th edn. Malden, MA: Blackwell.

Roberts, J. and Williams, A. (2004) Quality-of-life and asthma control with low-dose inhaled corticosteroids, *British Journal of Nursing*, 13(19): 1124–9.

Rodgers, J. (2000) Clinical pharmacological interventions in type 2 diabetes – the role of the nurse, *British Journal of Nursing*, 9(13): 866–70.

Rodgers, J. and Walker, R. (2002) NT plus: glycaemic control in type 2 diabetes, *Nursing Times*, 98(19): 56–7.

Scullion, J. (2005) A proactive approach to asthma, *Nursing Standard*, 20(9): 57–66, 68.

Shuttleworth, A. (2004) NT clinical: implementing new guidelines on epilepsy management, *Nursing Times*, 100(45): 28–9.

Simonson, T., Aarbakke, J., Kay, I., Coleman, I., Sinnott, P. and Lyssa, R. (2006) *Illustrated Pharmacology for Nurses*. London: Hodder Arnold.

Thomas, S. and MacMahon, D. (2002) Continuing professional development: Parkinson's disease – managing Parkinson's disease in long-term care, *Nursing Older People*, 14(9): 23–30.

Thomas, S. and MacMahon, D. (2004) Continuing professional development: Parkinson's disease, palliative care and older people – part 1, *Nursing Older People*, 16(1): 22–6.

Thomas, S. and MacMahon, D. (2004) Continuing professional development: Parkinson's disease, palliative care and older people – part 2, *Nursing Older People*, 16(2): 22–6.

Trounce, J. (2000) *Clinical Pharmacology for Nurses*, 16th edn. New York: Churchill Livingstone.

Wagstaff, S. (2004) Understanding the importance of effective glycaemic control, *Nursing Times*, 100(44): 45.

Wallymahmed, M. (2006) Insulin therapy in the management of type 1 and type 2 diabetes, *Nursing Standard*, 21: 50.

Watkins, P.J. (2003) *ABC of Diabetes*, 5th edn. London: BMJ Books.

Watkins, P.J., Amiel, S.A., Howell, S.L. and Turner, E. (2003) *Diabetes and its Management*, 6th edn. Malden, MA: Blackwell.

Wehrle, L. (2003) Epilepsy: its presentation and nursing management, *Nursing Times*, 99(20): 30–3.

Wolfe, S. (2006) Respiratory nursing: treatment of allergic rhinitis and asthma, *Nursing Times*, 102(20): 49–52.

Drugs used in mental health

8

Chapter contents

Learning objectives
Introduction
Anxiety
  The defence system
  The behavioural inhibition system
  Neurotransmitters in anxiety
Medicine management of anxiety
  Barbiturates
  Benzodiazepines
  Beta-adrenergic blockers
  Azaspirodecanediones
  Antipsychotics
  Antidepressants
Depression
  Key symptoms
  Ancillary symptoms
  Psychological factors
  Genetic factors
  Biological factors
    Hormonal influences

  The monoamine hypothesis
Medicine management
  of depression
  Tricyclic antidepressants
  Monoamine oxidase inhibitors
  Selective serotonin re-uptake inhibitors
  Other drugs
  St John's wort (Hypericum perforatum)
Psychosis
  Typical antipsychotics
    Mesolimbic pathway
    Tuberoinfundibular pathway
    Nigrostriatal pathway
  Atypical antipsychotics
  Side-effects
Case studies
Key learning points
Calculations
Multiple choice questions
Recommended further reading

Learning objectives

After studying this chapter you should be able to:

- Give an overview of the incidence of mental health problems in the UK.
- Define the term 'pathological anxiety'.
- List three major classifications of anxiety disorder.
- Explain how defence and behavioural systems contribute to anxiety.
- List two neurotransmitters thought to be implicated in anxiety.
- Explain in simple terms how benzodiazepines work.
- Outline the biological basis of depression.

- Give three examples of different groups of antidepressant drugs.
- Outline the mode of action of selective serotonin re-uptake inhibitors (SSRIs).
- Name two drugs used in bipolar depressive illness.
- Explain simply the biological basis of schizophrenia.
- List the positive and negative symptoms of schizophrenia.
- Give reasons why there are differences between typical and atypical antipsychotics.
- Give examples of typical and atypical antipsychotic drugs.
- Give reasons for the difference in side-effects between typical and atypical antipsychotics.

Introduction

The aim of this chapter is to introduce you to drugs used in common mental health problems. The chapter examines three key areas of mental health intervention:

- anxiety;
- depression;
- psychosis.

Mental health issues extend into all aspects of nursing and an appreciation of the range of medications and how they work is essential for today's nurses. One in four adults in the UK experience at least one diagnosable mental health problem in any one year, and one in six experiences this at any given time (Office for National Statistics 2001). It is estimated that approximately 450 million people worldwide have a mental health problem (World Health Organization 2001).

Anxiety

Anxiety is a fairly common, normal and usually self-limiting emotion, with which we are all familiar. For some people however, feelings of anxiety can be intolerable and can become disabling. This level of anxiety is considered to be pathological and requires prompt diagnosis and active treatment to help the sufferer regain and maintain their previously normal lifestyle. At this level, anxiety can manifest with wide and varied symptoms, both physical and psychological.

Anxiety is not simply one illness but a group of disorders characterized by psychological symptoms such as diffuse, unpleasant and vague feelings of apprehension, often accompanied by physical symptoms of autonomic arousal such as palpitations, light-headedness, perspiration, 'butterflies' and, in some patients, restlessness.

There are six main classifications of anxiety disorders:

1. panic disorder;
2. social phobia;
3. generalized anxiety disorder;
4. obsessive-compulsive disorder (OCD);
5. post-traumatic stress disorder (PTSD);
6. mixed anxiety and depressive disorder.

An understanding of the physiological mechanisms thought to be involved in the development of pathological anxiety is vital to ensure appropriate treatment of anxiety disorders. First it is important to understand that two brain systems appear to be involved in the generation of anxiety.

The defence system

The defence system controls our responses to danger. It receives stimuli related to the threat of danger and the brain interprets these stimuli and responds as required. The defence system is responsible for the so-called 'fear, fight or flight' responses. It can be a protective mechanism, whereby we can respond to threats or perceived threats and prepare the body to defend itself or to flee from the danger. It can also be activated by things which are not real threats, but are *perceived* as real by the anxiety sufferer and can become pathological.

The behavioural inhibition system

This system prevents a person from getting into danger and is responsible for *avoidance behaviour*. It is also involved in learning not to do dangerous things, therefore allowing future avoidance of anxiety-provoking situations. This can lead to anxiety sufferers withdrawing from real life situations because of the fear of being placed in danger, leading to agoraphobia, claustrophobia and social isolation.

Neurotransmitters in anxiety

The brain is a complex organ and with respect to anxiety many different neurotransmitters are involved. These include the following monoamines:

- noradrenaline (NA);
- 5-hydroxytryptamine (5-HT) or serotonin;
- gamma-aminobutyric acid (GABA).

The exact role these neurotransmitters play in anxiety is not fully elucidated, but using drugs that act on these systems can be beneficial in the management of anxiety.

Medicine management of anxiety

Although there is much commonality within the various anxiety disorders, it would be unwise to try to treat them all in the same way as they have important differences which necessitate variances in treatment. Anxiety management can be broken down into the following categories:

- **non-pharmacological:** psychological;
- **pharmacological:** single and combined psychotropic and non-psychotropic treatments;
- **combinations** of pharmacological and non-pharmacological treatments;
- **surgical**.

In reality the mainstay of anxiety treatment is pharmacological. Anxiolytic treatment should ideally be effective and quick-acting for rapid relief from the disabling symptoms. The treatment should not be too sedative as this can be as detrimental as the anxiety itself. This is achievable in the current pharmacological climate, but can often come at a price. The following drugs have all been used at one time to treat the symptoms of anxiety; many are still in use today:

- barbiturates;
- benzodiazepines;
- beta blockers;
- azaspirodecanediones;
- antipsychotics;
- antidepressants.

Barbiturates

Barbiturates are potentiators of the GABA-A receptor which has a *pentameric structure*. It has five sub-units which surround an ion channel which conducts chloride (Cl-) ions (see Figure 8.1). It is the major inhibitory neurotransmitter in the brain and central nervous system. Therefore potentiation of an inhibitory transmitter channel leads to increased inhibition, or reduced activity at the receptors the chloride ion acts on. This causes a 'dampening down' effect for all neuronal activity. When the Cl- ion channel is opened by GABA, the barbiturate drug molecule can enter the channel and causes it to remain open for a longer period of time than GABA alone would. This allows for more chloride from outside the neurone to enter it, so reducing the chance of an action potential being generated. This means that the barbiturate drugs cause a potentiation of GABA transmission and a reduction in neuronal activity.

There are downsides to using barbiturate drugs such as amobarbital (formerly amylobarbitone). They have a narrow therapeutic index, which means that the blood level of the drug needed for a beneficial effect is very close to the blood level which is toxic. This in turn means that it is easy to take too little and have no drug effect, or too much and reach toxicity. They also have addictive

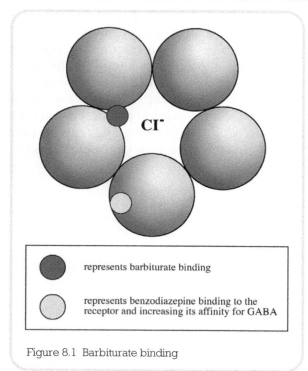

CI⁻

represents barbiturate binding

represents benzodiazepine binding to the receptor and increasing its affinity for GABA

Figure 8.1 Barbiturate binding

properties and patients can easily become dependent on them. They can also cause problems if taken with alcohol as it can increase their effects. For this reason they are very rarely used in anxiety management in modern times.

Benzodiazepines

For many years, the commonest and first-line pharmacological treatment for anxiety disorders was the prescription of a benzodiazepine drug. More recently this approach has changed with increased knowledge of the addictive and dependence problems and the abuse potential associated with benzodiazepines such as Diazepam and Temazepam. The use of these drugs has been related to significant long-term problems. The CSM issued the following advice which can be found in the BNF (2008: 55):

Benzodiazepines are indicated for the short-term relief (2–4 weeks only) of anxiety that is severe, disabling or subjecting the patient to unacceptable distress, occurring alone or in asso-

ciation with insomnia or short-term psychosomatic, organic or psychotic illness. The use of benzodiazepines to treat short-term 'mild' anxiety is inappropriate and unsuitable . . . benzodiazepines should be used to treat insomnia only when it is severe, disabling, or subjecting the individual to extreme distress.

All things considered however, benzodiazepines are still one of the most effective treatments for acute, transient anxiety. Like barbiturates, these drugs potentiate the effects of GABA but do so by a different mechanism. They bind to a specific benzodiazepine binding site (or receptor) which is situated on one of the sub-units of the GABA-A receptor. Their mechanism of action is to increase the affinity of GABA which leads to an increased ability and frequency of GABA to open the Cl- channel. Unlike barbiturates, benzodiazepines need GABA to be present all the time the channel is open, not just at activation, for them to have their effect. This makes them safer than barbiturates because they have a wider therapeutic index and less chance of toxicity and accidental overdose.

For use in anxiety, doses tend to be low, with higher doses being reserved for use in insomnia. This means that the side-effect of sedation should occur at a lower incidence although for some people drowsiness is a problem.

Another major side-effect of benzodiazepines is respiratory depression, and this should be monitored on initiation of therapy.

Clinical tip

When a patient starts taking a benzodiazepine it is very important that you warn them of the possible sedative effects and discuss the dangers of driving or operating heavy machinery.

Beta-adrenergic blockers

These drugs are used not to treat the central nervous system transmitters thought to be involved in anxiety, but to treat the *physical* symptoms that are often manifest in anxiety such as palpitations, tremors, sweating and shortness of breath. They will not affect the psychological aspects of anxiety, so the patient will still feel anxious.

There are many beta-blocking drugs, but only propranolol and oxprenolol are licensed for use in the management of anxiety. The use of these drugs may help people with mild anxiety to function in situations where before their symptoms would have proved problematic.

Clinical tip

If the patient also suffers from diabetes do not forget to warn them that taking a beta blocker may inhibit the normal signs and symptoms of a hypoglycaemic attack.

Azaspirodecanediones

Buspirone is the only drug in its class available for the treatment and management of anxiety symptoms. Its mechanism of action is not fully elucidated but it is known to affect the serotonergic receptors, inhibiting serotonergic transmission. This effect develops quickly but the anxiolytic effect does not typically occur for two to three weeks. This can be problematic in anxiety treatment as patients often cannot tolerate the delayed onset of action.

Buspirone is not associated with addiction or dependence, but is only licensed for short-term use, although it can be used for several months under specialist supervision.

Antipsychotics

There is evidence that certain antipsychotic drugs have positive benefit in the treatment and management of anxiety. The method by which they relieve anxiety is not known, but these drugs are associated with emotional changes and effects on symptoms such as agitation. In anxiety management they are used in doses much lower than would be needed for their antipsychotic effects. Drugs such

as haloperidol, flupentixol and tri-fluoperazine can be used as anxiolytics and have a quick onset. They are especially useful if the patient has a diagnosis of psychosis, as their anxiety may be related to this.

Like barbiturates and benzodiazepines, some of the side-effects of antipsychotic drugs can be compounded by alcohol.

Antidepressants

The tricyclic antidepressants (TCAs) have a positive effect in generalized anxiety disorder and panic disorder, although many of these drugs are not licensed for such indications. TCAs have been used in the past for mixed anxiety/depressive disorders but they do not appear to have a significant specific anxiolytic activity.

It may be that their anxiolytic effect is related to their sedative properties. It takes two to three weeks for the anxiolytic and antidepressant effect to develop, suggesting that the mechanisms for both are related.

Another type of antidepressant, selective serotonin re-uptake inhibitors (SSRIs) can appropriately be used in chronic anxiety of longer than four weeks' duration. Their mechanism of action is fully explained in the section on depression. The anxiolytic action takes two to three weeks to develop which is concurrent with the onset of antidepressant effect, again suggesting that the mechanisms are related. Some SSRIs have associated increased anxiety until the antidepressant effect occurs, and for this reason concomitant use of a benzodiazepine for the first two or three weeks is often recommended in anxiety, with a low starting dose of SSRI building up as tolerated.

Treatment is usually long term and often doses are at the higher end of the dosage scale for full effect. Examples of SSRIs in common use for anxiety are:

- fluoxetine and sertraline, licensed to treat anxiety symptoms accompanying depression and for OCD;
- fluvoxamine, licensed for the treatment of OCD;
- citalopram, licensed for the treatment of panic disorder;

- paroxetine, licensed for the treatment of social phobia, panic disorder, OCD and mixed anxiety and depression.

Depression

Depression is one of the most common serious psychiatric illnesses. Depressive or affective disorders involve a disturbance of mood or affect (cognitive and emotional symptoms), which are frequently associated with changes in behaviour, energy levels, appetite and sleep patterns (biological and physiological symptoms). Depression sufferers report a poor quality of life or morbidity. This often extends to their carers and can be detrimental to their close relationships. Depression has a high incidence of mortality which can often be due to suicide.

Depression can be:

- **Unipolar**, where the mood or affect is always low. This is characterized by misery, malaise, despair, guilt, apathy, indecisiveness, low energy and fatigue, changes in sleep patterns, loss of appetite and thoughts of suicide. It can be either *reactive* or *endogenous*. Reactive depression implies that the cause of the illness is brought about by severe stress. Endogenous depression on the other hand occurs when no obvious external causative factor can be identified.
- **Bipolar**, where the mood or affect and behaviour swing between depression and mania. This type of depression has a greater tendency to include an inherited component.

For a diagnosis of depression the patient must have certain key symptoms and also exhibit some ancillary symptoms. This assists the diagnosis and categorization of the depression.

Key symptoms
- Depressed mood.
- Inability to experience pleasure from normally pleasurable life events such as sex (anhedonia).
- Lack of energy.

Ancillary symptoms
- Changes in weight and appetite.
- Sleep disturbance.
- Low self-esteem.
- Psychomotor agitation or retardation.
- Guilt or self-reproach.
- Difficulty in concentrating.
- Suicidal thoughts.

Depression can be defined as mild, moderate or severe based on the number and incidence of these symptoms.

The aetiology of depression is still unclear. The biological theories relating to the disease would suggest that there are many factors in the development of depressive disorder including psychological, genetic, biological and neurochemical.

Psychological factors
These are known to play a part in the development of many types of depression and can be categorized as follows:

- Childhood and developmental experiences that are seen as negative, such as abuse, be it physical, mental or sexual; separation from one or both parents with maternal separation being particularly traumatic; breakdown of the relationship between parents and/or problems with the parent/child relationship.
- An unusually high number of what are termed as 'significant life events'. These are often ranked according to their perceived impact, with bereavement, especially of a spouse, topping the list. Surprisingly, 'positive' life events such as getting married or the birth of a baby also have a significant impact. This may be due to a major change in lifestyle.
- Stress which can be deemed as unusual or continual such as stress at work or in a relationship.
- The absence of a secure or confiding relationship. This can be particularly relevant to the elderly and those who have lost a loved one, and may also explain why those who live alone have a higher tendency to become clinically depressed.

Genetic factors

These are implicated in many areas of mental and physical health. Although no individual genes have yet been identified in depressive disease, there is a strong suggestion from family and twin studies of a genetic basis for a vulnerability to depression. A number of genes may be related to the function of known neurotransmitters and receptors, suggesting a biological effect. Other genes may be involved in influencing how a person perceives and responds to a certain kind of event or stressor, which may lead to depression in certain people but not in others.

Biological factors

Biological factors have become a major focus for research into depression and antidepressant drugs. Two distinct areas are implicated:

- hormonal influences;
- the monoamine hypothesis.

Hormonal influences

Cortisol, a corticosteroid, is known as the 'stress hormone' and has been linked to depression. Many people go on to develop depression if they are subjected to repeated and prolonged stress. Ongoing research is linking corticosteroids with monoamines to try to complete the picture.

The monoamine hypothesis

Many monoamines have been implicated in depression. Monoamines are, as their name suggests, organic compounds with a single (mono) amine group. They have the biological function of being neurotransmitters and neuromodulators and exert their effects at receptors located predominantly on neurones. They were first implicated as having a role in depression in the 1960s. This was due to the fact that the main antidepressant drugs used at that time (the TCAs and monoamine oxidase inhibitors, MAOIs) both have chemical actions on monoamines. It was suggested that reduced levels of monoamines could be a causative factor in depressive illness, although this hypothesis can be ar-

gued both for and against. Hence the monoamine hypothesis could explain why:

- drugs that deplete levels of monoamines are depressant in their nature (e.g. reserpine, methyldopa);
- drugs that increase the availability of monoamines *can* improve mood in depressed patients (e.g. TCAs and MAOIs);
- the concentration of some monoamines is notably reduced in the cerebrospinal fluid (CSF) of depressed patients.

But equally the hypothesis does not explain why:

- drugs that increase the availability of monoamines have *no effect* on mood in depressed patients (e.g. amphetamines, cocaine).
- some older antidepressants have no effect on monoamine systems (e.g. iprindole);
- there is a therapeutic delay of two weeks for the full effects of monoamine antidepressants to be seen.

Medicine management of depression

The BNF describes the main antidepressant drugs as shown in Box 8.1. We can now look at the mechanism of their action.

Tricyclic antidepressants

TCAs are powerful drugs which block the reuptake of two major monoamines, noradrenaline and serotonin, also known as 5-hydroxytryptamine (5-HT). This means that there is more of the monoamine available to the receptors and this has an antidepressant effect. However, drugs in this class, such as amitriptyline, act at other receptors which can lead to side-effects such as:

- **sedation**, which can be useful if the drug is taken at night and insomnia is a problem. Sedation can be increased if the drugs are taken with alcohol and this can be problematic;

Box 8.1 Antidepressants

Group	Abbreviation	Example
Tricyclic antidepressants	TCAs	Amitriptaline
Antidepressants related to TCAs		Trazodone
Monoamine oxidase inhibitors	MAOIs	Phenelzine
Reversible inhibitor of monamine oxidase-A	RIMA	Moclobemide
Selective serotonin re-uptake inhibitors	SSRIs	Citalopram
Other drugs	NARIs SNRIs AAAs	Reboxitine Venlafaxine Mirtazapine

- **cardiac rhythm problems**, which can be severe in overdose;
- **anticholinergic effects** produced by action at muscarinic receptors, such as urinary retention and constipation;
- **more seizures** in epileptic patients.

Clinical tip

Please remember to reassure the patient that side-effects of TCAs such as a dry mouth, blurred vision and becoming dizzy on standing (postural hypotension) are common. However, if the patient finds these intolerable they should make an appointment to discuss other drug options.

Monoamine oxidase inhibitors

Monoamine oxidase (MAO) exists in two forms, MAO-A and MAO-B, and both are responsible for chemically breaking down monoamines to render them inactive. MAOIs block this breakdown, and phenalzine is an example. The blocking leads to an increase in the availability of the monoamines which, as with TCAs, leads to an antidepressant effect.

These drugs are used infrequently due to their high risk of drug interactions, especially with other antidepressants. They are also able to interact negatively with some foodstuffs containing tyramine and dopamine (e.g. some cheeses, red wine, pickled herring and others). This interaction can cause blood pressure to increase to a dangerous level and patients on these medications are warned to avoid these foods.

MAOIs bind irreversibly but there is a reversible MAOI, moclobemide, which is also used.

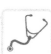

Clinical tip

You will not often encounter the use of MAOIs in clinical practice. However, if you do, please remember that the patient will need a treatment card. This will have information about diet, the taking of other medicines and the use of alcohol. The patient needs to be told to carry this card at all times and to show it to any doctor or dentist treating them.

Selective serotonin re-uptake inhibitors

This group of drugs act selectively at serotonin (5-HT) neurones to produce their antidepressant action. They have very similar profiles regarding their antidepressant effects and the main differences between them lie in their abilities to cause drug interactions and effects.

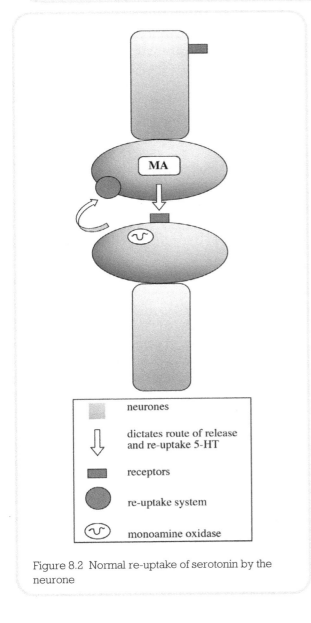

Figure 8.2 Normal re-uptake of serotonin by the neurone

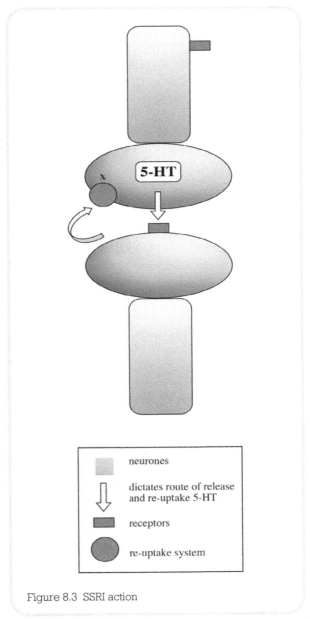

Figure 8.3 SSRI action

5-HT is released from the neurone into the synapse to have its action on receptors (see Figure 8.2). After release it is taken back up into the neurone that released it by a transporter located in the neuronal membrane. SSRIs inhibit the re-uptake of 5-HT from the synapse after it has been released. This leads to an increase in the amount of 5-HT present in the synapse available for action at receptors which respond to 5-HT and has an antidepressant effect (see Figure 8.3).

SSRIs have far less side-effects that other antidepressants and are safe in overdose. This makes them a good first-line choice of drug for treating most types of depression.

The main drugs prescribed in this class are Fluoxetine and Citalopram. The main reported side-effects include nausea and diarrhoea, loss of sexual desire and libido, some anxiety during initiation of treatment and occasionally sleep disturbances.

The effects of SSRIs take up to 14 days to fully develop and this should be explained to patients at commencement of treatment. The NICE guideline on the management of depression (2004) recommends the use of SSRIs. There is some evidence to suggest that, particularly in adolescence, SSRIs can increase the risk of suicide and self-harm. Any such risks should be balanced against the effectiveness of using these drugs in treating a patient's depression.

Clinical tip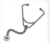

When prescribing SSRIs, doctors, nurses and pharmacists should warn patients of the possible risks of suicidal behaviour and monitor them closely in the early stages of treatment.

Other drugs

There are some other drugs that are useful in the treatment of depression. They include:

- **Flupentixol:** an antipsychotic drug which can be used to treat mild to moderate depression.
- **Mirtazapine:** an alpha adrenoceptor antagonist which is a relatively sedating antidepressant.
- **Reboxitine:** a noradrenaline specific re-uptake inhibitor.
- **Venlafaxine:** a noradrenaline and 5-HT specific re-uptake inhibitor which may have a quicker onset of action compared to noradrenaline or SSRIs alone.
- **Tryptophan:** a naturally occurring precursor to 5-HT which is obtained from our diet but can be given in its pure form. The theory is that if more of the precursor is available, the body will make more 5-HT, leading to an antidepressant effect. It can be used as an adjunct therapy with MAOIs and TCAs.

For bipolar depression, the treatment options are limited to lithium and some anticonvulsant drugs. Lithium treatment has been used for many

Box 8.2 Other drugs used in the treatment of depression

Drug class	Example
TCAs	Amitriptyline
MAOIs	Phenelzine
SSRIs	Fluoxetine
NARIs (noradrenaline reuptake inhibitors)	Reboxitine
SS/NARIs	Venlafaxine

years to prevent and treat bipolar depression. It is referred to as a 'mood stabilizer' as it helps to prevent the swings of mood (from depression to mania) typical of this type of illness. Lithium is a naturally occurring metallic element. Its action in the management of bipolar depression is poorly understood, but is thought to be linked to its actions on monoamine neurotransmission. It is however unclear how its actions relate to its therapeutic effects. It is a drug with a narrow therapeutic index and a long half life so it needs careful monitoring as there is a high risk of toxicity in overdose which can be fatal.

Clinical tip

It is important to remember that every patient taking lithium should be provided with a treatment card detailing the correct dose, blood test details and advice on drinking alcohol, taking other medicines and the effects of toxicity. When caring for someone who is taking lithium you should be aware of the need for monitoring the patient's fluid intake and also of the implications of sickness and diarrhoea. It is important that the patient avoids dehydration as this will increase the risk of lithium toxicity.

Some anticonvulsant medicines such as sodium valproate and carbamazepine have been found to have beneficial effects in bipolar depression. They are thought to be safer than lithium but are still associated with serious side-effects.

St John's wort (Hypericum perforatum)

Although not a drug prescribed for depression in the UK, St John's wort is worthy of a mention in this section. It is a popular herbal remedy, readily available for the management of mild forms of depression and used by many people. However, St John's wort can induce drug metabolizing enzymes in the liver which can lead to changes in how the body metabolizes other medications, causing interactions and side-effects. For this reason, the use of St John's wort with many medications is not recommended. The BNF section on interactions (Appendix 1) should be consulted for all patients taking St John's wort to ascertain its risk with other medicines. Interestingly, many of the drugs affected are conventional antidepressants. The concentration of active ingredients in St John's wort varies from preparation to preparation, making monitoring difficult.

When patients cease taking St John's wort there are concomitant changes in drug metabolizing enzyme performance and therefore a risk of drug toxicity.

Psychosis

Schizophrenia is the main psychotic mental health disorder because of its prevalence, its young age of onset (15–45 years) and its chronic and disabling nature. The pathophysiology is not completely understood but several theories have been postulated, including one linking dopamine to the condition. This has been strengthened by the fact that many drugs which are effective in schizophrenia act as dopamine receptors.

Schizophrenia is a disorder of thought and thought processes, perception, emotion and volition. Its symptoms fall into two main categories, positive and negative in character, which can include the following:

Positive:

- delusions;

- hallucinations;
- disordered thought.

Negative:

- poverty of speech;
- flattened affect;
- social withdrawal;
- anhedonia (inability to experience pleasure);
- apathy;
- attention deficit.

The distinction between positive and negative symptoms is important, as the main drug treatments tend to have most effect on positive symptoms, whereas negative symptoms are very hard to treat.

Other psychotic illnesses include:

- schizoaffective disorder;
- delusional disorders;
- some depressive and manic disorders.

Neuroleptic or antipsychotic medication is the mainstay of antipsychotic intervention. It has its actions on the dopaminergic system and receptors. It may take several weeks to have its full effect and these drugs are associated with many side-effects. The antipsychotic actions and extra-pyramidal side-effects of neuroleptic drugs are strongly correlated with their ability to block central dopaminergic transmission. The extra-pyramidal system is a neural network located in the brain that is part of the motor system involved in the coordination of movement. Antipsychotic drugs, by blocking dopamine receptors, can lead to a variety of movement disorders as a result of their effect on the extra-pyramidal system. This means that often, to obtain full control of the symptoms of schizophrenia, the doses used can cause increased side-effects. The ability of certain drugs to act on dopaminergic transmission and relieve the symptoms of psychosis was the basis of the dopamine hypothesis of schizophrenia first postulated in the 1960s.

Antipsychotic drugs are classified as typical or atypical in their actions. There are many dopamine receptors and other receptor types that are acted on by these drugs. Most typical antipsychotics act at D_2 receptors while most atypical antipsychotics act at D_1 and D_4 receptors. Having said this, most of these drugs have actions at other receptors as well, especially at higher doses and this is often what causes the side-effects.

A particular problem with taking antipsychotic medication daily is that certain patients may not see the need to continue taking the medicine. Quite often the patient has little understanding of their problem and as a result they may feel well and therefore decrease intake. Certain antipsychotic drugs are therefore given as what is known as a *depot injection*. This is an injection of a drug, usually given via the IM route, which releases its active compound in a consistent way over a long period of time. Depot injections are usually either solid or oil-based. The advantages of using a long-acting depot injection include increased medication compliance and a more consistent serum concentration. However, one significant disadvantage is that the drug is not immediately reversible since it is slowly released.

Clinical tip

When giving a depot injection you should use a 'Z track' injection method. This seals the medication deeply within the muscle and allows no exit path into the subcutaneous tissue and skin. This is accomplished by moving the skin and subcutaneous tissues by 2.5–3.75cm laterally, prior to the injection, and immediately releasing the same tissues after the injection.

Examples of typical and atypical antipsychotic drugs are listed in Box 8.3.

Typical antipsychotics

Typical antipsychotics are associated with more side-effects despite their good antipsychotic action, due to their actions at the D_2 receptors. They are structurally similar and chemically related. The actions at D_2 receptors can be viewed in terms

Box 8.3 Drugs used in the treatment of psychosis

Typical	Atypical
Chlorpromazine	Sulpiride
Promazine	Clozapine
Flupentixol	Olanzapine
Haloperidol	Quetiapine
Trifluoperazine	Risperidone

of the three main pathways they influence (see Figure 8.4):

1 the mesolimbic pathway;
2 the tuberoinfundibular pathway;
3 the nigrostriatal pathway.

Mesolimbic pathway
This is associated with the psychological effects of these drugs:

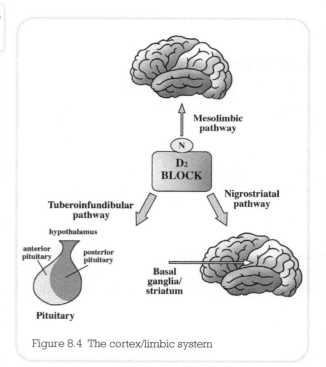

Figure 8.4 The cortex/limbic system

- antipsychotic effects;
- sedation;
- impaired performance.

Tuberoinfundibular pathway

This is associated with neuroendocrine effects of these drugs:

- **hyperprolactinaemia:** this is a high blood level of prolactin from the pituitary gland which can cause production of breast milk as well as menstrual/erectile problems;
- **amenorrhoea:** the absence of periods in a woman of reproductive age;
- **galactorrhoea:** the spontaneous flow of milk from the breast;
- **gynaecomastia:** this is enlargement of male breast tissue;
- **infertility:** this is the biological inability of a man or a woman to contribute to conception.

Nigrostriatal pathway

This is associated with movement disorders produced by these drugs:

- **Parkinsonism:** characterized by lack or slowness of movement, muscular rigidity and tremor;
- **dystonia:** characterized by sustained muscle contractions causing twisting or repetitive movements, or adoption of abnormal postures;
- **akathisia:** characterized by restlessness and unease;
- **tardive dyskinesia:** characterized by abnormal involuntary movements of the face.

Clinical tip

As a nurse it is important that you are an advocate on behalf of the patient. This means reporting any signs and symptoms of any medication to senior colleagues or the medical staff. This will ensure side-effects can be dealt with early.

Atypical antipsychotics

These drugs, unlike the typical antipsychotics, share very little similarity in structure or chemistry.

- **Clozapine** is a dibenzodiazepine neuroleptic and exerts its effect via dopamine receptors but also acts at muscarinic and 5-HT receptors.
- **Sulpiride** is a dopamine and 5-HT blocker and is effective in the treatment of schizophrenia. It is suggested that sulpiride has more action at mesolimbic dopamine receptors.
- **Risperidone** has a higher affinity for 5-HT than dopamine and a lower incidence of sedation and extra-pyramidal side-effects at low doses than other neuroleptics.

Clinical tip

Clozapine carries the risk of lowering the agranular white blood cell count (agranulocytosis), therefore monitoring of blood levels of neutrophils is a mandatory condition of treatment. As these blood cells protect us from infection it is important that the level does not drop significantly. You should be aware of patients on this medication that complain of relatively minor ailments such as repeated sores.

Side-effects

The side-effects of typical antipsychotics occur because of the actions at a variety of receptors, including the dopamine receptors which are responsible for their beneficial effects. Antipsychotics are associated with a high level of side-effects, some of which are quite severe in their nature and are commonly referred to as extra-pyramidal side-effects (EPSEs). Examples are:

- **Dopaminergic side-effects** such as acute neurological effects (dystonia, Parkinsonism) and chronic neurological effects (tardive dyskinesia, tardive dystonia).

- **Neuroendocrine side-effects** such as amenorrhoea, galactorrhoea and infertility.
- **Idiosyncratic side-effects** such as neuroleptic malignant syndrome. This is a life-threatening reaction that some people have to antipsychotic medicines.
- **Cholinergic side-effects** such as dry mouth, blurred vision, constipation, urinary retention, ejaculatory failure.
- **Histaminergic side-effects** (sedation).
- **Adrenergic side-effects** such as hypotension, arrhythmia.
- **Miscellaneous side-effects** such as photosensitivity, heat sensitivity, cholestatic jaundice, retinal pigmentation.

Management of these side-effects is often necessary by prescription of other drugs to reduce their severity. These drugs can be grouped as follows:

- **Anticholinergics**, used for motor side-effects (e.g. benzhexol, procyclidine).
- **Psychostimulants**, used in demotivation.
- **Benzodiazepines**, used for akathisia (e.g. lorazepam).
- **Beta blockers and antihistamines**, occasionally used for akathisia.

Atypical antipsychotics in general have a much better side-effect profile and are generally better tolerated and safer to use.

Clinical tip

Often the first sign of neuroleptic malignant syndrome is a fever. Therefore you should be observant and report any changes in the temperature of an individual who has just commenced their medication regimen.
If treated early this condition does not have to be fatal.

Clinical tip

Atypical antipsychotics are far from being free of side-effects. You should warn patients that on certain drugs weight gain can be a significant problem. Also, secondary type II diabetes is becoming a problem associated with taking atypical antipsychotics and you may be involved in screening patients by urine testing or carrying out random blood glucose measurements.

Case studies

① Debbie Butcher is a well educated 37-year-old woman with two previous episodes of depression in the last 10 years, both of which were treated. The first (post-natal depression) was treated with Fluoxetine for one year and the second (reactive to her ninth miscarriage) with Citalopram for two years. The doctor has prescribed her another SSRI and she asks you to explain how it works.

- How would you describe the mechanism of action of SSRIs, with particular reference to onset of action and the monoamines involved?

② Anil Khan is a 53-year-old man who has been diagnosed with schizophrenia since the age of 23. He has been cared for in a number of institutions and has recently been admitted to an independent mental health hospital. For many years he has been treated with a variety of typical antipsychotics, and the medical staff suggest he is drug resistant and are trying him on the newer atypical therapy.

- How would you describe to a junior nurse the actions of such drugs on the individual?
- How would you explain the differences between the two types of antipsychotic medication?

Key learning points

Introduction

➢ One in four adults in the UK experience at least one diagnosable mental health problem in any one year.

➢ There are some 450 million people worldwide with a mental health problem.

Anxiety

➢ Anxiety can become intolerable for some people and is therefore considered to be pathological.

➢ It is a group of disorders characterized by both physical and psychological symptoms.

➢ There are six main classifications.

➢ Our defence mechanism can become stimulated by perceived threats.

➢ Avoidance behaviour can be initiated.

➢ A number of neurotransmitters are involved (e.g. noradrenaline).

➢ Anxiolytic treatment should be effective and quick-acting.

Medicine management of anxiety

➢ Barbiturates potentiate GABA.

➢ They have a low therapeutic index.

➢ They have addictive properties.

➢ They are rarely used in anxiety management.

➢ Benzodiazepines are still one of the most effective treatments for acute and transient anxiety.

➢ They also potentiate the effects of GABA.

➢ These drugs have a wider therapeutic index and are therefore less toxic than barbiturates.

➢ Beta-adrenergic blockers are used to treat the physical symptoms of anxiety.

➢ They may help people with mild anxiety to function in certain situations.

➢ Buspirone is the only azaspirodecanedione in its class used in the treatment of anxiety.

➢ It has effects on serotonin receptors but takes a number of weeks to achieve an anxiolytic effect.

➢ Some evidence exists to suggest that antipsychotics may have a positive benefit in the treatment of anxiety.

➢ How they relieve anxiety is not known and they are only used in low doses.

➢ Drugs such as haloperidol and flupentixol may be used.

➢ Antidepressants such as tricyclic compounds seem to have an effect in generalized anxiety disorder.

➢ SSRIs can appropriately be used in chronic anxiety (e.g. fluoxetine).

Depression

➢ Depression is the most common serious psychiatric illness.

←

➤ Has a high incidence of morbidity.
➤ Unipolar depression is characterized by a continuous lowering of mood.
➤ Bipolar disorder is characterized by a swinging of mood between depression and mania.
➤ Depression is characterized by certain key symptoms such as lowering of mood, sleep disturbance and changes in weight and appetite.
➤ The aetiology is still unclear but is thought to include psychological factors, genetic factors and biological factors.
➤ A variety of neurotransmitters (monoamines) have been implicated in the causation of depression.

Medicine management of depression

➤ TCAs affect the re-uptake of noradrenaline and serotonin.
➤ Side-effects include sedation, anticholinergic effects and cardiac dysrhythmias.
➤ MAOIs work by stopping the body breaking down neurotransmitters such as serotonin.
➤ These drugs are now infrequently used due to the high risk of drug interactions.
➤ SSRIs act selectively at serotonin neurones.
➤ Serotonin is increased at the synapse.
➤ SSRIs have less side-effects and are safer in overdose compared to other antidepressants.
➤ Venlafaxine is a drug that has a quick onset and raises the levels of noradrenaline and serotonin available to the body.
➤ Bipolar depression is treated with lithium or certain anticonvulsant drugs.
➤ Lithium needs careful monitoring as it can cause toxicity.
➤ Drugs such as sodium valproate and carbamazepine have also been found to be beneficial in the treatment of bipolar disorder.

Psychosis

➤ Schizophrenia is the main psychotic mental health disorder.
➤ Positive symptoms include delusions, hallucinations and disordered thought.
➤ Negative symptoms include social withdrawal, flattened affect and apathy.
➤ Drugs used in the treatment of schizophrenia block the actions of dopamine in the brain.
➤ Typical antipsychotics are associated with more side-effects.
➤ Typical antipsychotics block the three main dopamine pathways.
➤ Typical antipsychotics produce side-effects which are often described as being extrapyramidal.
➤ Atypical antipsychotics include clozapine, sulpiride and risperadone.
➤ Atypical antipsychotics in general have less severe side-effects, are tolerated better and are safer to use.

Calculations

1   A client is prescribed 50mg of amitriptyline and 25mg tablets are available. How many tablets will you give?

2   A client is prescribed 300mg of promazine and 100mg tablets are available. How many tablets will you give?

3   A client is prescribed 100mg of promazine and 25mg tablets are available. How many tablets will you give?

4   A client is prescribed 1.25mg of clonazepam and 0.5mg tablets are available. How many tablets will you give?

5   A client is prescribed 20mg of haloperidol decanoate by intramuscular injection and 50mg in 1ml of liquid for IM injection is available. How many ml will you administer?

6   A client is prescribed 5mg of flupenthixol decanoate by IM injection and 40 mg in 2ml of liquid for IM injection is available. How many ml will you administer?

7   A client is prescribed 5mg of haloperidol orally and 2mg in 1ml of syrup is available. How many ml will you administer?

8   A client is prescribed 10mg of promazine orally and 50mg in 5ml suspension is available. How many ml will you administer?

9   A client is prescribed 4g of trifluoperazine orally and 5g in 5ml liquid forte is available. How many ml will you administer?

10 A client is prescribed 2.5mg of promethazine hydrochloride orally and 5mg in 5ml of elixir is available. How many ml will you administer?

Multiple choice questions

Try answering these multiple choice questions to test what you have learned from reading this chapter. You can check your answers on page 202.

1 Depression can be described as

a) Unipolar and multipolar
b) Multipolar and oligopolar
c) Oligopolar and bipolar
d) Bipolar and unipolar

2 SSRI drugs act on which monoamine?

a) Adrenaline
b) Dopamine

←

c) Serotonin
d) Noradrenaline

3 Benzodiazepines bind to which receptor complex?

a) NA
b) DA
c) BDZ
d) GABA

4 Neuroleptic medications are used for

a) Psychosis
b) Neurosis
c) Epilepsy
d) Parkinson's disease

5 Lithium can be described as

a) A mood enhancer
b) A mood reflector
c) A mood inducer
d) A mood stabilizer

6 5-hydroxytryptamine is also known as

a) Buscopan
b) Serotonin
c) Adrenaline
d) 5-BC

7 Amylobarbitone is an example of

a) A barbiturate
b) A benzodiazepine
c) A tricyclic
d) An SSRI

8 Which of the following is a benzodiazepine?

a) Benzopine
b) Tazepam
c) Diazepam
d) Lazypram

9 How long does it take until SSRI antidepressants begin to have a therapeutic effect?

a) The same day
b) Two to three weeks
c) One month
d) Six days

10 Psychotic symptoms can be

a) Positive and additive
b) Negative and additive
c) Positive and negative
d) Negative and cumulative

For further assistance with calculations, please see Meriel Hutton's *Essential Calculation Skills for Nurses, Midwives and Healthcare Practitioners* (Open University Press 2009).

Recommended further reading

Beckwith, S. and Franklin, P. (2007) *Oxford Handbook of Nurse Prescribing*. Oxford: Oxford University Press.

Brenner, G.M. and Stevens, C.W. (2009) *Pharmacology*, 2nd edn. Philadelphia, PA: Saunders Elsevier.

Clayton, B.D. (2009) *Basic Pharmacology for Nurses*, 15th edn. St. Louis, MO: Mosby Elsevier.

Coben, D. and Atere-Roberts, E. (2005) *Calculations for Nursing and Healthcare*, 2nd edn. Basingstoke: Palgrave Macmillan.

Downie, G., Mackenzie, J. and Williams, A. (2007) *Pharmacology and Medicines Management for Nurses*, 4th edn. Edinburgh: Churchill Livingstone.

Gatford, J.D. and Phillips, N. (2006) *Nursing Calculations*, 7th edn. Edinburgh: Churchill Livingstone Elsevier.

Karch, A.M. (2008) *Focus on Nursing Pharmacology*, 4th edn. Philadelphia, PA: Lippincott Williams & Wilkins.

Lapham, R. and Agar, H. (2003) *Drug Calculations for Nurses: A Step-by-step Approach*, 2nd edn. London: Arnold.

NICE (National Institute for Health and Clinical Excellence) (2004) *Clinical Guideline 23: The Management of Depression in Primary and Secondary Care*. London: NICE.

Office for National Statistics (ONS) (2001) *Psychiatric Morbidity Report*. London: ONS.

Simonson, T., Aarbakke, J., Kay, I., Coleman, I., Sinnott, P. and Lyssa, R. (2006) *Illustrated Pharmacology for Nurses*. London: Hodder Arnold.

Trounce, J. (2000) *Clinical Pharmacology for Nurses*, 16th edn. New York: Churchill Livingstone.

World Health Organization (WHO) (2001) *The World Health Report 2001: Mental Disorders Affect One in Four People*. Press Release WHO/42, 28 September. Geneva: WHO.

Patient concordance

9

Chapter contents

Learning objectives
Introduction
Adherence, compliance and concordance
Factors influencing effective medicine use and concordance
Patient awareness of need for medication
Patient awareness of consequences of *not* taking medication
Time of dosing
Side-effects
Product formulation
Product packaging

Interactions with other medication
Ability to obtain prescription
Confusion or agitation states including memory impairment
Patient empowerment in chronic disease management
Patient education
Patients as partners in decision-making
Case studies
Key learning points
Calculations
Multiple choice questions
Recommended further reading

Learning objectives

After studying this chapter you should be able to:

- Articulate the meaning of adherence, compliance and concordance with regard to the taking of medication.
- Discuss the factors that influence effective medicine use and concordance.
- Outline the salient points a nurse must consider in assessing, planning, implementing and evaluating patient education with regard to medicines.
- Describe how a patient with a chronic disease may be empowered to manage their medication.
- Explain how patients may become partners in medicine management.

Introduction

Medicines that are prescribed but not taken by patients represent a large loss in drug and prescribing costs and an enormous waste of expensive health professionals' time. In 2007 the National Audit Office estimated that about £100 million is wasted each year on medication dispensed but returned to pharmacies. The aim of this chapter is to introduce the reader to the concepts of adherence, compliance and concordance with respect to medicine management. Nurses need to have an understanding of pharmacology at a level which will allow them to inform and educate the patients in their care. Without effective information and education surrounding their medications, many patients are unable to understand the need for them to take their medications as prescribed to ensure optimum drug performance.

Adherence, compliance and concordance

Much of the time, we use the terms *adherence*, *compliance* and *concordance* almost interchangeably, when in fact they each have quite different and specific meanings.

Adherence has a dictionary definition that suggests sticking to something. When we talk about patients adhering to their medication regimen we quite literally mean: are they sticking to the prescribed instructions for taking their medication? For a patient to adhere to their medication regimen, they need very little information from the prescriber. They attend a consultation and present the prescriber with a problem or symptom. The prescriber makes a diagnosis, prescribes the medication and the patient is issued with a prescription to take for dispensing. Information needs to be given verbally to the patient about how to take their medication, and printed instructions are issued with their drugs. The patient needs to read the instructions or follow the prescriber's guidance and adhere to that. The knowledge gained from the information given should make the reasons for adherence clear to the patient. The prescriber should

also consider aspects of the medication regimen that may make adherence difficult for the patient and factor them into any decision-making. This adherence may seem an obvious thing for patients to do, but patients frequently, and for many reasons, take their medication in a manner other than the instructions with which they were issued with by the prescriber. Non-adherence to medication regimens can have serious consequences, depending on the medication being prescribed. Failure to adhere is, not surprisingly, a particular problem in the management of chronic illness, especially when the patient does not feel ill. Some of the drug therapies covered in Chapter 7 of this book like asthma, diabetes and hypertension incur especially high levels of non-adherence and it is common for patients to alter or abandon taking their drugs.

Compliance with a medication regimen differs from the act of simply adhering to it. By complying with the prescriber's instructions the patient automatically adheres to the medication regimen. But compliance suggests that information is given to allow the patient to make the *choice* to comply. There is some involvement of the patient in the medication regimen, but compliance relies largely on the patient following the prescriber's recommendations. Some patients do not like the term 'compliant' as it suggests that if they diverge from the regimen, they are seen as non-compliant, a negative term.

Concordance is where the patient–prescriber relationship surrounding medication regimens is seen to be more equal in footing and there is a current initiative to further involve patients in the treatment process and so improve their compliance and adherence. This requires an active participation by the patient, and a confident and self-aware prescriber or medicines educator. Concordance involves the sharing of knowledge, understanding and beliefs by both parties. The prescriber offers their knowledge and expertise of the condition to be treated and the range (if appropriate) of treatment options available, be they pharmacological or non-pharmacological. The prescriber then provides information about the medicines to be considered including any cautions, contraindications and side-effects. This gives the patient an *informed choice*. Patients bring their knowledge of their lifestyle and practices to the equation. This can include work patterns, social, religious and cultural aspects, and practicalities, such as an ability to open medicine bottles. This can help the prescriber to narrow the range of prescription options available. By good knowledge-sharing and communication an effective decision as to the most appropriate medicine to be prescribed can more easily be reached and the result is likely to improve concordance and compliance. It could be argued that all of this should happen in the adherence model and for many patients it does. The goal is ultimately for the patient to take their prescribed medicine in the most effective way in order for their condition to improve. In 2009, NICE published guidance on medicines adherence which is concerned with enabling patients to make informed choices by involving and supporting them in decisions about prescribed medicines. At this time it is the most up-to date resource for prescribing in the UK.

Factors influencing effective medicine use and concordance

There are many factors which can influence a patient's ability to adhere, comply or demonstrate concordance when it comes to medications. Non-compliance and non-adherence may be an intentional act on behalf of the patient or may be an involuntary act of which they are not even aware. Both can often be associated with the amount and quality of education and information given by the prescriber, dispenser and administrator of the medication at the time treatment is initiated. It may be that the impact of the medication regimen on the patient's daily routine is intolerable to them. They may not be able to take the medication as prescribed or even attend to the filling of their prescription. It may equally be that they feel that by taking the medication in a way other than prescribed by the doctor, they are exerting control over the situation to improve, in their minds, the likely outcome.

The main factors to consider can be summarized as follows:

- patient awareness of need for medication;
- patient awareness of consequences of *not* taking medication;
- time of dosing;
- side-effects;
- product formulation;
- product packaging;
- interactions with other medication;
- ability to obtain prescription;
- confusion or agitation states including memory impairment.

Patient awareness of need for medication

It is important that patients are fully aware of the need for them to take their medication. This may seem an obvious statement, but in some cases patients do not want to take medication, and if they are not fully cognizant of the need for the medication, non-adherence can occur. This can be especially true in patients who have received a diagnosis when they had not been feeling unwell. An example is when a condition is picked up on routine screening (e.g. raised blood pressure). The importance of taking antihypertensive medication should be explained thoroughly and the prescriber should also outline the consequences of not taking the medicine.

Patient awareness of consequences of not taking medication

This is perhaps more important than the reasons *for* taking medication. Patients' perceptions of the benefits and risks of taking medication have been shown to influence compliance. Using the example of high blood pressure, there are many consequences of not taking antihypertensive medication. The continual presence of a raised blood pressure increases the patient's risk of stroke and heart attack, both of which can lead to premature death. It cannot therefore be understated how important good information and education are in this area.

Time of dosing

This can be very important for some patients. A good example is antibiotic prescriptions. Some schools will not administer medications to children during school hours but insist on a parent coming in to give the medicines. For a child who is prescribed antibiotics three or four times per day and is well enough to attend school, necessitating dosing during school hours, this can be problematic. It could lead to the child being kept off school, the parent missing work or the antibiotics being taken inappropriately. It may be prudent therefore to consider prescribing an antibiotic that can be taken once or twice daily that can be appropriately administered around school hours.

Side-effects

Intolerable side-effects are one of the main reasons for non-compliance with medicine regimens. No drug is completely free from side-effects, but some effects are tolerable for some patients but may not be for others. Information and education about potential side-effects is vital in medicines management. If a patient experiences side-effects it may lead to them stopping the medication and possibly not seeking advice from the prescriber. A good example here is Citalopram, an antidepressant medication which can cause nausea as a side-effect. This nausea is usually transient and will pass after about two weeks, hence it is important to educate the patient about this, as most people can put up with a mild side-effect for a short period if they know it will pass, and they will continue with the medication.

Some side-effects can be severe and may even become adverse for the patient if left unchecked. It is very important to stress to patients that if they experience any side-effects they should seek advice at once.

Product formulation

In some cases, the simple formulation of the medication makes adhering to the regimen difficult if not impossible. Children are an important group to consider from this point of view. Many children under the age of 10 have great difficulty in swallowing tablets, so liquid medicine is the preferred choice. Some children, especially smaller children, will also dislike the taste of their medicine. If this is analgesia, it is worth the parent trying different brands, as they can be obtained in different flavours to help them find a product suitable for their child.

In inflammatory bowel disease the use of rectal medication can be a cause for concern. For some patients rectal medication is unacceptable and produces anxiety regarding the route of administration. Even with a clear educational plan of action, to expect a patient to use medication that produces such anxiety may be unrealistic. This issue should be thoroughly explored with the patient before treatment is prescribed.

Product packaging

The elderly or those with manual dexterity problems can often have trouble with product packaging. The main problem is child-proof caps on medicine bottles, but some blister packs can prove difficult to get into as well. Dispensing pharmacies are able to help with this if asked. Tablets can be supplied in bottles with normal caps on request. Medication can also be supplied in easy-to-open packs.

Interactions with other medication

Although patients may be taking their medication as prescribed, it is important to consider other medication or specific instructions on timing of dosing. Some drugs are not fully absorbed from the stomach if they are taken at the same time as an antacid preparation. Some should be taken with food, others after food and still others before food, so it is important that the patient takes their medicines exactly as prescribed to ensure optimum effect.

Ability to obtain prescription

For some elderly or infirm patients this could be a hurdle to medication adherence. If the patient cannot physically go to the pharmacy to collect their prescription, it follows that they cannot take the medication. This has become much less of a problem as a result of initiatives by some pharmacies to collect prescriptions, issue the medication and deliver it to the patient's home. Many community pharmacies offer this service and will collect repeat prescriptions direct from the doctor's surgery. It is important that patients are made aware of this service where it exists.

Obtaining a prescription for some people may start with the priority of which medications they can afford. Not all people who require a large number of medicines get help in paying for them. Some people in employment who have to pay for their prescriptions ration themselves to those medications that they perceive to be the most important or most obviously efficacious. The 'lesser' medications (in the patient's eyes) may not be purchased.

Confusion or agitation states including memory impairment

If patients who suffer from agitation states and/or memory impairment are on several different medications, their condition in itself can cause problems in terms of adherence and compliance. Multi-dose boxes and dated boxes are available and can be made up by pharmacies for all the medicines needed. Such boxes have a strip for each day, with time to take the medication highlighted. This allows patients to see whether or not they have taken their medication. In more severe cases, patients may need family or carers to administer their medicines.

Forgetfulness is a major cause of non-compliance. Patients should be taught behaviour strategies such as reminders, self-monitoring tools, cues and reinforcements. The use of aids, such as the dosette box, should not be viewed as just having a use for older people, but for those with unstructured or hectic lifestyles such as the young.

Patient empowerment in chronic disease management

Patients who suffer from long-term or chronic diseases often want to be empowered in the management of their conditions, and this can include the choice and modification of any medications

prescribed. They can feel despondent about having to take medication for life, and naturally want the medication to treat their condition with minimal impact on their lifestyle and routine. More and more patients want to be involved and to feel in control of their disease, rather than it controlling them. Education and information is the key in patient empowerment. Education allows patients to develop a knowledge and understanding of their disease and its management, and is sometimes equivalent to that of the health professional involved in their care. There is a wealth of sources of information for patients. The internet and its many search facilities have dramatically opened up the amount of information available, however there can be problems with accessing the internet. In areas of low socioeconomic status, access to global information may become entangled with economics and therefore inequalities in medicine information almost certainly exist.

For patients not able to access the internet, information can be provided by leaflet format, or by attendance at 'help' groups, often formed for many chronic diseases. This is no substitute for good information provided by health care professionals, but can serve to augment that information.

Patient education

This should be individualized to the patient and is an important component of nursing care. Patients should have an individualized medication programme as part of their discharge plan. The nurse should provide the patient with medication leaflets to promote recall of details given to them during any medication teaching. Before teaching patients, nurses should plan what the session aims to achieve and what the outcomes of the session should be. When developing a teaching plan, nurses should allocate time to discuss with patients what they would like to know about their medication. Do not forget that some patients are very knowledgeable about their condition and the medicines that they take. Therefore it is important not to be patronizing and to seek out the patient's level of knowledge prior to undertaking an educational role. The importance of the nurse understanding aspects of pharmacology is paramount. This is why you need to carry on increasing your knowledge in this area.

Once patients leave hospital other members of the primary care team have a duty to continue a more long-term education plan with regard to their medicines. Primary care specialists, GPs and pharmacists should be involved in information-giving and evaluation of the patient's level of concordance. This is especially important with elderly people as the medication regimens in this group tend to be complex.

Patients as partners in decision-making

Except when patients are in hospital, it is they who have to manage their own medication. Ironically it is often patients themselves who remain passive when it comes to consulting with health care professionals about their medicine management and behavioural changes. It is a relatively new concept for us to consider the patient as a partner in any decision-making process with regard to the management of their care, let alone bringing medication into the arena. This is, however, the main factor to consider in promoting concordance. The good consultation skills of a health care professional should always include the patient at all stages of the consultation. Patient trust and cooperation can enhance the information obtained by the health care professional which subsequently improves the outcome of the session.

Many patients want to be active partners in decision-making and this should be encouraged. People are often more likely to take their medication if they can hear themselves putting forward solutions. Therefore, asking patients' views, listening and helping them think the problem through and make a decision is more effective than *telling* them what to do.

Listening skills are important in information exchange so that both parties can think about and reflect on each other's viewpoint. The nurse needs to be aware of verbal and non-verbal cues which may indicate that the patient is becoming reluctant or defensive. Such a reaction usually means that the approach taken by the nurse is making the pa-

tient feel uncomfortable. The nurse therefore must develop an increased level of sensitivity and understanding of the interaction taking place.

It is however essential that the partnership is *functional*. Some patients feel that because this is *their* disease *they* will make the decisions. This can lead to an inappropriate balance in the partnership and may be detrimental, with the knowledge and expertise of the health care professional not being acknowledged.

Some patients do *not* want to be active partners in decision-making, and their wishes should not be ignored. Many patients come to see their doctor with a symptom or problem, want the doctor to make a diagnosis and prescribe treatment. They respect the doctor's knowledge and expertise and many feel that 'doctor knows best'. This attitude actually requires more skill on behalf of the prescriber who, in order to most appropriately prescribe, requires information about lifestyle and practices that will enable them to make a more informed decision.

Relapse is common, so the need for open discussion is extremely important. All nurses need to acknowledge that it is possible that a patient may want to stop or change their medication.

A number of psychological models have been developed in order to understand health behaviours relevant to compliance. The most popular model is the *health belief model* which puts forward the view that health-related behaviours or the seeking of health interventions depend on four factors:

1. **perceived susceptibility** (the person's assessment of their risk of getting an illness);

2. **perceived severity** (the person's assessment of the seriousness of the illness, and what this could mean for them);

3. **perceived barriers** (the person's assessment of any influences which may discourage the adoption of health-related behaviours);

4. **perceived benefits** (the person's assessment of the beneficial outcomes of adopting a health-related behaviour).

Another popular model is called the *theory of planned behaviour*. This focuses on the attitudes and intentions of the patient in relation to performing certain health behaviours. The theory suggests that the intention of the person to perform a compliant act depends on their attitude, subjective pressure and perceived levels of being controlled by others.

Often these models are adopted by nurses and others in an attempt to empathize with the patient and to ensure a positive outcome to health education. Both models rely on what psychologists call the *locus of control*. This refers to a patient's belief about what causes the positive or negative outcomes in their lives, particularly in specific areas like health. Some people have what is known as an *internal locus of control*, which means that the person believes that they have the ability to control changes in their lives. The opposite is an *external locus of control* where the person believes that they have little or no control and that their life circumstances have been dictated by factors external to them.

As we have discussed, how patients perceive themselves is important in planning care and treatment options. Successful concordance with medication has a higher likelihood if there is an understanding of why a patient may or may not adopt a given behaviour. From this we can see that changing health attitudes is an area that requires much understanding from the nurse. We must seek to see the patient's perspective and understand what taking medications means to that individual. Without this knowledge, any attempt at promoting concordance will be at best transitory and superficial.

Case studies

① Kubi Garise is a 75-year-old woman who suffers from rheumatoid arthritis, hypertension, and has the early symptoms of dementia, especially memory problems. She is on medication for her arthritis and hypertension, but also takes aspirin daily and a drug to protect her stomach. She lives alone and is only mobile around her house and garden. Her family are worried that she may not be taking her medication properly.

■ Can you identify strategies to improve her compliance?

② Ella Jenkins is 4 years old and needs antibiotics for an ear infection. Her mother is struggling to get her to take the medicine the doctor has prescribed as she does not like the taste. Mrs Jenkins has decided not to give the medicine as she does not like upsetting Ella.

■ How would you go about educating Mrs Jenkins as to the importance of complying with the medication?

■ What suggestions could be made to the prescriber to help improve the likelihood of Ella taking her antibiotics?

Key learning points

Introduction

➤ Nurses need a sound knowledge of pharmacology to inform health promotion.

←

Adherence, compliance and concordance

➢ Adherence to a medication regimen is sticking to the prescribed instructions for the taking of medication.
➢ Compliance involves the patient making some choices based on information given by the prescriber.
➢ Concordance involves the sharing of knowledge, understanding and beliefs by both the prescriber and the person taking the medicine.

Factors influencing effective medicine use and concordance

➢ Non-compliance and non-adherence may be an intentional act or an unintentional act by the patient.
➢ It is important that patients are fully aware of the need to take their medication.
➢ The patient must be aware of the consequences of not taking their medication.
➢ Lifestyle and the timing of a dose are important.
➢ Considering the side-effects a medicine has on a person is of paramount importance.
➢ How the product is formulated may have an impact on whether a person will take the medicine or not.
➢ Product packaging can be troublesome for people with limited dexterity.
➢ Other medications that the person is taking need to be assessed to ensure drug interactions are prevented.
➢ Even the ability of a person to obtain the prescription itself can be an obstacle.
➢ People who suffer from confusion or other cognitive impairments have special requirements.

Patient empowerment in chronic disease management

➢ Include the patient in choice of medication and any modifications to their medicines.
➢ Enable the patient through internet access and self-help groups.
➢ Each patient should have an individual plan.
➢ Use educational leaflets to reinforce the knowledge base of the patient.
➢ Draw up learning objectives and consider how you will evaluate what has been taught.
➢ Good consultation skills should always include the patient.
➢ Problems in the patient–prescriber relationship lead to poor decision-making.

Calculations

1 A doctor has prescribed 0.25mg of digoxin. You have 125 microgram tablets. How many should you give?
2 How many grams are in 2.5kg?

3 You have a vial of actrapid containing 100 units per ml. How much do you need to give 12 units?

4 How many micrograms are in 1.25g?

5 You have a bottle of amoxicillin syrup containing 250mg in 5ml. How much do you need to give 125mg?

6 You have a vial of gentamycin containing 80mg in 2ml. How much do you need to administer 100mg?

7 A patient is being given an IV infusion, and is to receive 1 litre of fluid over five hours. What volume of fluid in ml will they receive each hour?

8 How many milligrams are in 0.1kg?

9 Given that w/v (weight to volume) = number of grams in 100ml, you have a solution of glucose 50 per cent w/v. How many grams of glucose will you have in 50ml?

10 Given that w/v (weight to volume) = number of grams in 100ml, you have a solution of sodium 30 per cent w/v. How many grams of sodium would be in 1000ml?

Multiple choice questions

Try answering these multiple choice questions to test what you have learned from reading this chapter. You can check your answers on page 203.

1 Adherence in drug therapy is defined as

a) Sticking to a medicines regimen
b) Commencing a medicines regimen
c) Stopping a medicines regimen
d) Monitoring a medicines regimen

2 Concordance should be aimed for

a) In patients on four or more medicines
b) In chronic disease management
c) In all patients prescribed medicines
d) Only in patients who have prescription-only drugs

3 Patient partnership in prescribing

a) Can only work in patients with a health care background
b) Helps promote concordance
c) Can only be achieved in hospital settings
d) Is inappropriate with children

←

4 Concordance is best achieved when

a) The doctor makes the prescribing decisions
b) The nurse makes the prescribing decisions
c) The patient makes the prescribing decisions
d) All of the above

5 Concordance can be affected by

a) The drugs prescribed for the patient
b) The patient's understanding of the medicines
c) The cost of the medications
d) How often the patient attends the surgery

6 Patients being provided with information on their medicines

a) Is the main responsibility of the prescriber and the pharmacist
b) Is the responsibility of the patient and the nurse
c) Is the responsibility of the prescriber only
d) None of the above

7 What route of administration of drugs is likely to have the best compliance?

a) IV
b) IM
c) Rectal
d) Oral

8 Non-compliant patients should always

a) Be advised to find a new doctor
b) Have their medicines changed
c) Be given help and information regarding their medicines
d) Have their medicines given by another route

9 The best way to promote concordance is

a) Information and cheaper drugs
b) Education and free prescriptions
c) Cheaper drugs and easier medicines regimens
d) Easier medicine regimens and education

10 Non-compliance with medicines regimens is

a) Restricted to the elderly
b) A potential problem for all prescribers
c) Not a problem in children
d) Avoidable only in well-educated patients

Recommended further reading

Badger, F. and Nolan, P. (2006) Concordance with antidepressant medication in primary care, *Nursing Standard*, 20(52): 35–40.

Banning, M. (2004) Enhancing older people's concordance with taking their medication, *British Journal of Nursing*, 13(11): 669–74.

Beckwith, S. and Franklin, P. (2007) *Oxford Handbook of Nurse Prescribing*. Oxford: Oxford University Press.

Brenner, G.M. and Stevens, C.W. (2006) *Pharmacology*, 2nd edn. Philadelphia, PA: Saunders Elsevier.

Clayton, B.D. (2009) *Basic Pharmacology for Nurses*, 15th edn. St Louis, MO: Mosby Elsevier.

Coben, D. and Atere-Roberts, E. (2005) *Calculations for Nursing and Healthcare*, 2nd edn. Basingstoke: Palgrave Macmillan.

Downie, G., Mackenzie, J. and Williams, A. (2007) *Pharmacology and Medicines Management for Nurses*, 4th edn. Edinburgh: Churchill Livingstone.

Ekman, I., Schaufelberger, M., Kjellgren, K., Swedberg, K. and Granger, B. (2007) Standard medication information is not enough: poor concordance of patient and nurse perceptions, *Journal of Advanced Nursing*, 60(2): 181–6.

Gatford, J.D. and Phillips, N. (2006) *Nursing Calculations*, 7th edn. Edinburgh: Churchill Livingstone Elsevier.

Karch, A.M. (2008) *Focus on Nursing Pharmacology*, 4th edn. Philadelphia, PA: Lippincott Williams & Wilkins.

Lapham, R. and Agar, H. (2003) *Drug Calculations for Nurses: A Step-by-step Approach*, 2nd edn. London: Arnold.

Matthews, E. (2004) Reflective practice: concordance with pain medication, reflection on an adverse incident, *British Journal of Nursing*, 13(9): 551–5.

Newell, K. (2006) Concordance with asthma medication: the nurse's role, *Nursing Standard*, 20(26): 31–3.

NICE (National Institute for Health and Clinical Excellence) (2009) *Clinical Guideline CG76: Medicines Adherence: Involving Patients in Decisions About Prescribed Medicines and Supporting Adherence*. London: NICE.

Simonson, T., Aarbakke, J., Kay, I., Coleman, I., Sinnott, P. and Lyssa, R. (2006) *Illustrated Pharmacology for Nurses*. London: Hodder Arnold.

Trounce, J. (2000) *Clinical Pharmacology for Nurses*, 16th edn. New York: Churchill Livingstone.

Willis, J. (2000) Patient compliance, *Nursing Times*, 96(35): 36–7.

Legal and professional issues

10

Chapter contents

Learning objectives

Introduction

The correct patient

The correct medicine

The correct dose

The correct site and method
   of administration

Covert administration
   of medicines

Mental capacity and competence in consent

Alteration of medicines

Reporting of drug errors

Controlled drugs

Supply and administration
   of medicines

Prescribing law and non-medical prescribing

Case studies

Key learning points

Multiple choice questions

Recommended further reading

Learning objectives

After studying this chapter you should be able to:

- Discuss the importance of identifying the correct patient as part of administering a medication.
- List the issues that are important in giving a patient the correct medicine.
- Describe the steps you would take in order to accurately calculate a drug dosage.
- Outline why it is important to recognize the correct route of administration when giving a drug.
- Discuss legal and professional dilemmas concerning giving a medicine in a covert manner.
- Explore the issues relating to a nurse crushing or tampering with a drug prior to its administration.
- Describe why it is important that nurses report any errors in the giving of medication.
- Describe the procedure a nurse has to undertake when giving a controlled drug.
- Demonstrate an understanding if what is meant by the term 'patient group directions'.
- Discuss the history of nurse prescribing.
- List the Acts that have led to nurse prescribing.
- Describe what is meant by the terms 'supplementary' and 'independent' prescriber.

Introduction

The aim of this chapter is to introduce you to the legal and professional issues faced by nurses in medicines management. Nurses are bound by the code of conduct laid out by the Nursing and Midwifery Council (NMC). The NMC has specific standards for administration of medication which must be adhered to. In addition, nurses are governed by the legislation surrounding medicines.

Administration of medicines is a skill that you will be exposed to during your pre-registration education. It is most important that you become involved in this procedure, so that you can become confident and competent as a practitioner. On your placements you need to be assertive in requesting to be involved in the administration of medicines because qualified nurses often carry out this task without necessarily involving the student.

Medicines are used for their therapeutic effects and careful administration of these is paramount. As a result, a number of legislative and professional standards are in place so that mistakes do not occur. In 2008 the NMC set out its latest guidance for the administration of medicines. This guidance highlights the importance of identifying the correct patient, the correct drug, the correct dose, the correct site and method of administration and the correct procedure. This chapter will use this framework to explore certain legal and professional issues that may arise during your initial education. The chapter will conclude by briefly exploring the future of the nurse's role in medicine management.

The correct patient

It is essential that you are aware of the relevant details of the person you are about to give a medicine to. For example, you need to know some background on the patient even before correctly identifying them. The first question that you might ask is whether the individual has the capacity to consent. This will be dealt with later in the chapter. You also need to consider the patient's diagnosis and physical capabilities. An area addressed in previous chapters is also important to consider at this

point: the question of hypersensitivity and allergies. There may also be special instructions that are important to remember such as whether the patient is to be kept nil by mouth.

At some point you will be working in a busy acute setting where the turnover of patients is high. In this environment it is unlikely that you will get to know patients very well and the safest way to identify a patient before giving them a medicine is by checking their wrist band (identity band). This band should contain accurate details that correctly identify the wearer.

Between November 2003 and July 2005 the National Patient Safety Agency (NPSA) received 236 reports of patient safety incidents and cases of 'near-misses' relating to missing wristbands or wristbands with incorrect information. Over the period February 2006 to January 2007 the NPSA received 24,382 reports of patients being mismatched to their care. We accept that not all these incidents involved the giving of medication but what these statistics highlight is the importance of thoroughly checking the identity of a patient.

You should find that 'core patient identifiers' are on their wristband, such as surname, forename, date of birth and NHS number. In long-term settings you may also find that photographs of patients are provided on their charts to help ensure that problems of misidentification do not occur.

The correct medicine

Most medicines have two names, the generic approved name (e.g. diazepam) and the proprietary or manufacturer's brand name (e.g. Valium). As a student one of your first tasks is to learn both the generic and proprietary (brand) names. On placement you will find that most health care professionals refer to drugs by their generic name whereas patients often refer to the brand name. The fact that drugs have more than one name makes the potential for error greater.

Prescription charts have to be written up using the drug's generic name, so limiting the chance for error. However, stocks of drugs on the wards and patients' individual drug boxes carry *both* names. You must make sure that when you are checking a drug you are satisfied it is the drug that is named on the prescription sheet. Most nurses would probably agree that medication packaging can be quite misleading and the names that are given to medicines can look and sound very similar. If you are in doubt please ask.

You must make sure you can read the name of the drug clearly, both on the prescription chart and on the packaging it is being dispensed from. You must *never* transfer drugs from one container to another, nor be tempted to agree to a drug being dispensed from a container which has had the label defaced or altered in some way.

When administering medicines to a patient it is also part of the nurse's responsibility to ensure that the drug is *appropriate* for the patient. Knowledge of the patient's medical history and their medical diagnosis is the main way of determining this, as is discussion with the prescriber and the patient. A patient should only be prescribed a medicine where there is a clinical need, and where non-pharmacological methods have proved insufficient.

Some medicines may be prescribed to a patient for a reason not under the drugs licence remit. This is not abnormal and discussion with the prescriber can reassure the nurse prior to administration that the drug is appropriate. A good example is that of amitriptyline. This drug is well known for treating depression but in more recent times has been prescribed in low doses to alleviate chronic back pain.

The correct dose

Another reason why drug errors occur relates to the potential for overdosing or under-dosing the prescribed medicine. As a nurse the NMC suggests that it is not enough for you to be able to give a drug but that you should have some understanding of *what* you are giving. Administering a medicine should not be a case of mechanically following a set of instructions but rather an intellectual event that is carried out thoughtfully. When you are involved in the procedure of medicine administration it is good practice to have an understanding of the drug's actions, interactions and side-effects. It is no defence to simply agree with the giving of the

medicine because you trust the doctor or the nurse. You must ensure that you use the BNF in any circumstances where you are unsure. All care settings that dispense drugs must have a copy on hand as a reference for all staff members. Find out where it is kept and make use of it during your placements. Make use of Appendix 1 covering interactions. Some patients are prescribed many medications for multiple conditions so it is important to be aware of any interactions between prescribed and OTC medicines, for example. Many drug combinations may have interactions which are of little or no clinical relevance, but others may have interactions with potentially serious or hazardous consequences. The ultimate responsibility lies with the prescriber, but the pharmacist involved in dispensing medicines and the nurse who administers medicines also have a role in identifying potential interactions for patient safety.

Our advice to you is to learn about a small number of drug groups which you come across regularly on your placement. If you do this for all the placements you visit over your three years you can build up a comprehensive portfolio of information and knowledge.

A number of authors in recent nursing literature suggest that errors occur in medicine administration because of a lack of basic mathematical skills in nurses themselves. Some writers even suggest that pre-filled infusion bags, electronic drip counters and user-friendly drugs such as single-dosed heparin injections all contribute to the deskilling of nurses in terms of their mathematical abilities.

It is true to say that this phenomenon has been recognized by nurse education and steps are being taken to remedy the situation. Since 2000 there has been a drive to increase student nurses' basic numerical skills. Part of the aim of this book has been to emphasize the importance of calculating accurate doses and to give you the opportunity to practise your maths outside the clinical setting.

In promoting safe practitice, some nurses have called for a greater use of, and emphasis on, calculators within practice settings. However, there is a counter-argument here that suggests we should use calculators *less* in practice. The thinking behind this is that calculators will become a substitute for the nurse using basic arithmetic. As a student nurse I am sure you will get your fair share of theoretical sessions on numeracy in nursing as part of your pre-registration education. The testing of basic levels of numeracy has now become part of the criteria for entry onto nurse education programmes. If you have not engaged in the calculation exercises in this book we believe you are missing out on a critical area of your knowledge. Most of the questions we have posed are basic in nature and are only included to give you a foundation. However, it is important that we all start somewhere, and the self-testing element of the book gives you an opportunity to get it wrong without undue criticism or pressure.

In practice we suggest that when involved in working out drug calculations you should:

- take *time* to work out your calculations;
- always *recheck* your answers;
- do not be rushed by colleagues or be embarrassed to tell them that you get a different answer; answers that look wrong probably are and it might be useful to make an initial logical estimate to base your final calculation on;
- if you are unsure do *not* be tempted to avoid losing face by simply agreeing for agreeing sake – this is dangerous.

The correct site and method of administration

You will probably have heard the one about the student nurse being asked to give a patient an aminophylline suppository to help their breathing. The sister came back five minutes later to find the student trying to insert the suppository into the patient's nose! Joking apart, you should be aware of which route the medicine is to be given. To simply ask for a medicine to be given by injection is not specific enough. As you are aware, there are a number of ways in which a drug could be injected: SC, IM or IV.

Recently, a person suffering from leukaemia was receiving regular chemotherapy by IV infusion. A junior doctor, by error, decided to give the medication into the person's epidural space and subsequently killed them. This situation would have to be dealt with under criminal law and a coroner would be involved. Less extreme examples of getting routes of administration wrong could be the difference in giving a medication sublingually instead of buccally. For example, a drug called glyceryl trinitrate, when prescribed buccally, should be placed under the top lip; but if prescribed sublingually it will be placed under the tongue. Medicines are designed and formulated to be absorbed according to the route of delivery; therefore, getting the route of a drug right is of paramount importance.

Covert administration of medicines

Administration of medicines covertly is a highly contentious issue in nursing. For example, to administer a medicine covertly to a capable adult would, in law, be looked upon as *trespass*. This is because the person receiving the medicine would not have consented. The Human Rights Act (1998) describes the need for nursing care to be given with respect and to be proportionate to the needs of the patient.

For a person to give consent, they need to have the mental capacity to understand an explanation, be able to make some form of choice and be able to communicate. Every person with mental capacity has a right to refuse medication if they so wish.

In exceptional circumstances, the law accepts that the giving of medicine to a patient unable to give consent is acceptable provided that the carer is acting in the best interests of the patient and that the care given is of a reasonable standard. Courts have also accepted that doctors may treat patients without their consent if it is seen to be in the best interests of that patient. There are obviously situations in nursing where consent has to be given by those other than the patient – for example parental responsibility, which includes the right to consent on behalf of children.

Where a patient lacks capacity, the law in England does not currently allow others, for example relatives, to give consent on someone's behalf without legal intervention. When dealing with somebody who does not have the capacity to give consent, professionals must rely on the principle of *necessity*. This means that treatment should only be given when it is necessary for the patient's health and well-being. However, relatives and carers are likely to have a detailed understanding of the patient's circumstances and can offer insights into what their best interests are. Therefore, the nurse should work in partnership with relatives and partners in order to provide the best care for the individual.

Despite the legal and professional debate, you may still come across patients having medicines hidden in their food or drink. Some authors suggest that this is still a common problem and is particularly prevalent in nursing homes. As a student nurse and future professional you should not engage in giving medication covertly to patients unless under exceptional circumstances.

Mental capacity and competence in consent

For those deemed unable to give consent due to lack of mental capacity, prior legal addressing of this situation can give relatives or carers the ability, in law, to act in the best interests power of attorney and power of welfare.

The Mental Capacity Act (2005) is designed to protect those who can't make decisions for themselves or lack the mental capacity to do so. The Act's purpose is:

- to allow adults to make as many decisions as they can for themselves;
- to enable adults to make advance decisions about whether they would like future medical treatment;
- to allow adults to appoint, in advance of losing mental capacity, another person to make decisions about personal welfare or property on their behalf at a future date;
- to allow decisions concerning personal welfare or property and affairs to be made in the best

interests of adults when they have not made any future plans and cannot make a decision at this time;
- to ensure an NHS body or local authority will appoint an independent mental capacity advocate to support someone who cannot make a decision about serious medical treatment, or about hospital, care home or residential accommodation, when there are no family or friends to be consulted;
- to provide protection against legal liability for carers who have honestly and reasonably sought to act in the person's best interests;
- to provide clarity and safeguards concerning research in relation to those who lack capacity.

The Act should only be used when the patient is unable to give consent for themselves and has been judged by a medical professional to be lacking in capacity.

When it comes to children and young adults, it is lawful for doctors to provide advice and treatment without parental consent providing certain criteria are met. These criteria, known as the Fraser Guidelines, require the professional to be satisfied that:

- the young person will understand the professional's advice;
- the young person cannot be persuaded to inform their parents;
- the young person is likely to begin, or to continue having, sexual intercourse with or without contraceptive treatment;
- unless the young person receives contraceptive treatment, their physical or mental health, or both, are likely to suffer;
- the young person's best interests require them to receive contraceptive advice or treatment with or without parental consent.

Although these criteria specifically refer to contraception, the principles are deemed to apply to other treatments, including abortion. Although the judgement in the House of Lords that produced these criteria referred specifically to doctors, it is considered to apply to other health professionals, including nurses.

If a person under the age of 18 refuses to consent to treatment, it is possible in some cases for their parents or the courts to overrule their decision. However, this right can be exercised only on the basis that the welfare of the young person is paramount.

Alteration of medicines

Sadly, few nurses are aware of the pharmacological dangers to the patient and of the legal implications of tampering with drugs.

Drugs only have a licence to be administered in the form in which they are packaged. Therefore, crushing tablets or separating capsules can alter the delivery system. This in turn will affect the pharmacokinetics and dynamics of the medicine resulting in changes in the speed of absorption and therapeutic efficacy.

A nurse who administers a medicine in a way that falls outside the product licence undertakes a degree of liability for any adverse effects caused by maladministration. The nurse can take steps to lessen any personal liability when giving a drug outside its product licence, and one reasonable step is to get the medication prescribed in an alternative form such as a liquid. Some companies specialize in making drugs in liquid form. It is most important, if you see a patient struggling to take medication in tablet or capsule form, that you inform the nurse in charge so that they can speak to the medical staff and get the prescription changed. A further precaution would be to discuss the crushing of the medicine with the pharmacist and get written approval from them that the practice is appropriate.

The issue of tampering with or crushing tablets is a particular dilemma when giving drugs enterally. Enteral feeding refers to the delivery of a complete nutritional feed directly into the stomach, duodenum or jejunum. This type of feeding is usually considered for malnourished patients, or in patients at risk of malnutrition who have a functional GI tract but are unable to maintain an adequate or safe oral intake. In your placement you may come across a variety of methods of giving enteral feeds,

for example, nasogastric (NG) or percutaneous endoscopic gastrotomy (PEG).

While tampering with or crushing medication is not a preferred method of administration it is likely that this has to happen when giving drugs enterally, especially if they are not available in liquid form. The nurse may crush or separate capsules as long as the doctor is aware that the drugs are to be given by this route. The doctor could then prescribe the drugs enterally, therefore making administration lawful. The problems of this type of administration becoming unlawful stem from tampering with the medicine but not informing the prescriber of this practice. Some clinical areas have developed separate protocols for enteral administration of medicines. When working in a hospital setting, informing the pharmacy regarding this route of administration is usually enough – they will then facilitate the drugs being available in an appropriate form. You will find that all hospitals have their own medicines policy which usually contains information on crushing or tampering with medicines. You need to become familiar with this document when you are in the placement area.

Reporting of drug errors

In its advice to nurses the NMC highlights the importance of an *open culture* in practice with regard to the reporting of drug errors. This needs to be fostered in order to encourage the immediate reporting of errors or incidents in the administration of medicines.

Unfortunately, as we work in a more and more litigatious society, drug errors are often not viewed on a case by case basis and disciplinary action is frequently taken against nurses for their mistakes. It could be argued that by taking this approach all that is being achieved is to make nurses reluctant to report such incidents.

As a student nurse, if you make a mistake you are not seen as being culpable in law. However, you need to learn from your mistakes. Therefore, if you make a drug error you may be asked to complete a *critical incident analysis* of what went on. Using this as a reflective tool you can identify risk management issues that you should have

Schedule	Drug example	Conditions
1	Cannabis	Possession and supply prohibited unless under Home Office rule
2	Morphine	Full controlled drug restriction, register required
3	Barbiturates	Special prescription requirements
4	Benzodiazepines	Minimal control, no safe custody, records required
5	Codeine	Minimal control, no safe custody, record-keeping less stringent than schedule 4

Table 10.1   Misuse of Drugs Regulations (2001) five schedules

developed in order to minimize the likelihood of the error occurring. The reflective analysis allows you to revisit the situation and to explore your reasons for the course of action you took. This can then be compared with the medicines policy to inform you of the importance of adhering to such important documents.

The adaptation of a no-blame culture is more conducive to the reporting of drug errors. It is a duty of care to the patient that you report any errors to the person in charge of your placement area. If you have seen an error occurring you *must* report it. This can be very difficult as a student because you want to fit into the team, and you might find yourself in the position of being a 'whistle-blower'. However, to ignore the incident is a breach of the legal duty of care that you owe to the patient. You would also be failing to follow the standards set in law for the safe administration of medicines.

Controlled drugs

There is much legislation surrounding the prescription, supply, storage and administration of medications. The Misuse of Drugs Act (1971), which supersedes the Dangerous Drug Act (1967), prohibits certain activities in relation to controlled drugs in terms of manufacture, supply and possession. The Act outlines three classes into which the medications it controls fall: class A (e.g. morphine); class B (e.g. codeine) and class C (e.g. buprenorphine).

The Misuse of Drugs Regulations (2001) define the classes of person who are authorized to supply and possess controlled drugs in a professional capacity and under set conditions. The activities governed are import and export, production, supply, possession, prescribing and record-keeping. The Regulations lay out five schedules defining the drugs included (see Table 10.1).

You will find that controlled drugs are stored in a particular way, being kept in a separate cupboard. You will often find that this locked cupboard is kept within another locked cupboard. The keys for the controlled drugs cupboard should be kept separate from other keys and the nurse in charge should keep these on his or her person while on duty. When you work on wards in hospital settings you will find that a warning light is placed on the outer cupboard. This indicates to staff whether the cupboard has been left open. No other items should be placed in the controlled drugs cupboard.

When giving a controlled drug you will find that a separate drug register is kept. This keeps an ongoing tally of the amount of drugs used and also lists all the patients that the drugs have been administered to, along with the date and time of administration.

When giving a controlled drug a particular procedure must be followed. This involves two people, one of which must be a qualified nurse or doctor. Some Trusts ask for *both* nurses to be qualified. Nevertheless, try to get involved in the administration of this category of medicine to gain a full understanding of the procedure and the nurse's role.

Before administering the controlled drug it must be checked against the amount last entered in the controlled drugs register. Once you have removed the drug from the controlled drug cupboard you must lock the cupboard and prepare the drug for administration. Once the drug has been administered you will have to detail in the controlled drug register the date, time, patient name, amount of drug given, who gave the drug, who witnessed the drug being given, and finally the new stock balance. You may also be involved in checking the stock of controlled drugs at a ward level. This is carried out on a regular basis. Please get yourself involved in this aspect of medicines management.

The ordering of a controlled drug is carried out using a specially designed order book. Controlled drugs can only be ordered by the nurse in charge. The pharmacy will have a copy of that person's signature which helps them to decide to dispense the drug or not.

Finally, when the controlled drug is delivered to the setting it is usually contained in a locked box and/or delivered by a designated person. The person collecting the drugs from the pharmacy has to sign for them and then someone signs to say they have been received in the clinical area. On receipt, the drugs are checked by two nurses, one of whom must be qualified, and signed for. The newly-ordered drugs are then entered onto the controlled drugs register by both nurses and the tally of drugs is amended accordingly.

Supply and administration of medicines

Traditionally nurses were only involved in administering medication. However, under certain circumstances, they are now involved in supply and administration of medications, usually under a Patient Group Direction (PGD). PGDs are written instructions for the supply or administration of medicines to homogenous groups of patients who require the same treatment. PGDs are used in situations where there is an advantage for patient care without compromising safety. In 1998, the *Supply and Administration of Medicines Under Group Protocols* report was published (DH 1998). This provided the legal framework for PGDs.

The PGD must be signed by the senior doctor or senior pharmacist involved in developing the direction. The legislation specifies that each PGD must contain the following information (see the Medicines and Healthcare Products Regulatory Agency at www.mhra.gov.uk/Howweregulate/Medicines):

- the name of the business to which the direction applies;
- the date the direction comes into force and the date it expires;
- a description of the medicine(s) to which the direction applies;
- class of health professional who may supply or administer the medicine;
- signature of a doctor or dentist, as appropriate, and a pharmacist;
- signature by an appropriate organization;
- the clinical condition or situation to which the direction applies;
- a description of those patients excluded from treatment under the direction;
- a description of the circumstances in which further advice should be sought from a doctor (or dentist, as appropriate) and arrangements for referral;
- details of appropriate dosage and maximum total dosage, quantity, pharmaceutical form and strength, route and frequency of administration, and minimum or maximum period over which the medicine should be administered;
- relevant warnings, including potential adverse reactions;
- details of any necessary follow-up action and the circumstances;
- a statement of the records to be kept for audit purposes.

Prescribing law and non-medical prescribing

Traditionally, doctors prescribed, pharmacists dispensed and nurses administered medication. Changes in legislation and the extension of health professionals' roles has seen this alter in recent years. The idea of prescribing other than by a doctor was first suggested in 1986 following a review of community nursing services, leading to a report by Baroness Julia Cumberlege. In this report, *Neighbourhood Nursing: A Focus for Care* (DHSS 1986) it was concluded that much of a district nurse's time was being wasted in obtaining prescriptions for basic dressings and appliances required for patient care. The report also detailed the frustration of some nurses involved in palliative care at not being able to vary timing and dosage of prescribed analgesics as dictated by the patient's condition.

Further review by Dr June Crown (DH 1989) and her advisory group began the revolution in prescribing practice. Her initial suggestions included:

- 'initial prescribing' from a restricted formulary;
- supply within an agreed clinical protocol;
- amendment of timing and dosage of medicines prescribed previously within a patient-specific protocol.

It was a further five years before the first nurse began prescribing. The Medicinal Products: Prescription by Nurses Act was passed in 1992 and nurse prescribing was made legal in 1994 when secondary legislation came into force. Now suitably qualified district nurses were able to prescribe from a limited formulary for specific clinical conditions.

For nurses, however, these changes did not go far enough in addressing their need to prescribe for their patients. They found the formulary restrictive and in some cases were not able to prescribe appropriately for the patients in their care. The *Review of Prescribing, Supply and Administration of Medicines* (DH 1999) took nurse prescribing further and described two different groups of prescriber: the *dependent prescriber*, now known as the *supplementary prescriber* and the *independent prescriber*, who was a doctor or a dentist.

It was suggested that the dependent prescriber would be able to prescribe certain medications following initial assessment and diagnosis of the patient by the independent prescriber and the development of an agreed clinical management plan (CMP). This allowed nurses access to many more medications as long as they were stated on the CMP.

By now, other allied health professionals were in roles that would benefit from them being able to prescribe. The Health and Social Care Act 2001 (Section 63) allowed the extension of prescribing rights and privileges to certain health care professionals. Changes to the 'Prescription Only Medicines Order' and NHS regulations gave suitably qualified nurses and pharmacists supplementary prescribing rights in April 2003 (DH 2005).

This was extended to chiropodists/podiatrists, radiographers, physiotherapists and optometrists in May 2005 and allowed the government to help meet targets set in the *NHS Plan* (DH 2000). It led to increasing flexibility among multidisciplinary teams by empowering staff and providing efficient and timely access to medicines and an increased patient choice.

Further reviews by the Department of Health (DH) enabled nurses and pharmacists to prescribe independently of a CMP from 2006. These autonomous practitioners are responsible for assessment, diagnosis and treatment of patients for whom their clinical conditions fall within that area of competence. They can prescribe from the whole BNF, with only some restrictions surrounding controlled drugs and non-licensed medications.

Nurse prescribers must have an identified prescribing role within their area of practice, be at least three years post-registration and have successfully completed an approved programme of training. This allows additional registration with the NMC as a nurse prescriber, with the nurse following guidelines and standards laid out by their governing body.

It is envisaged that there will be further developments in the field of nurse prescribing, and although it is not expected that student nurses will become prescribers, they must be aware of who can prescribe to safely participate in medicines management as part of their role.

Case studies

① As a student nurse you are accompanying a staff nurse on a drug round. Mr Ajani has been prescribed paracetamol but the drug prescription chart has not been signed by a doctor. The staff nurse asks you to give the medicine to the patient, saying she will get it signed later. Look at the NMC standards for medicines management, and review the implications for yourself and the staff nurse if you administer this medication.

② You are accompanying a district nurse on a patient home visit. The nurse is a prescriber and can prescribe paracetamol for Mrs Simpson (age 66) under a CMP.

■ Using supporting literature from the internet, what conditions must the nurse have satisfied to become a prescriber? Reflect on the holistic care of this patient with the nurse being a prescriber and compare it to the differences in Mrs Simpson's care if the nurse were not able to prescribe.

Key learning points

Introduction

➤ Medicines are used for their therapeutic effects and careful administration of these is paramount.
➤ The NMC has set out guidance for the administration of medicines.
➤ There are legal and ethical principles to consider when administering a medicine.

The correct patient

➤ Capacity to consent is an important issue.
➤ Checking for allergies is also important.
➤ You need to identify that you have the correct patient before giving a medicine.

The correct medicine

➤ Drugs generally have at least two names: generic and brand.
➤ Prescription charts are written using the generic name.
➤ Being able to read clearly the name of the medicine on the prescription chart and on the packaging is important.

The correct dose

➤ Overdosing and under-dosing of patients is a problematic area.
➤ Using the BNF is imperative in drug administration.
➤ Nurses' basic arithmetic has been criticized for drug errors.
➤ Practise calculating medicine doses when you are on placement.

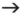

←

The correct site and method of administration

➤ Drugs can be given by a number of routes.
➤ It is important that you correctly identify the correct route.
➤ Drugs are designed to be delivered by the correct route.

Covert administration of medicines

➤ Covert administration of a medicine to a capable adult is seen as a trespass in law.
➤ Consent is an important area of drug administration.

Mental capacity and competence in consent

➤ Mental capacity to consent is an issue for children and vulnerable adults.

Alteration of medicines

➤ Drugs must not be crushed or tampered with.
➤ Altering the delivery system of a medicine is outside its licence.
➤ Alteration of a drug will affect its pharmacokinetics and dynamics.
➤ You will not be able to predict side-effects if you alter a drug.
➤ Involve the pharmacy department if a patient is having problems taking the medication in its prescribed format.
➤ Giving a medicine in an unlicensed manner is unlawful.

Reporting of drug errors

➤ An open no-blame culture is important in the reporting of drug errors.
➤ Student nurses are not culpable in law for errors.
➤ If you are involved in a drug error or if you see a drug error being made you must report it.
➤ If you make a drug error you should work through a reflective critical incident analysis in order to learn from your mistakes.

Controlled drugs

➤ The Misuse of Drugs Act (1971) prohibits certain activities in relation to controlled drugs.
➤ The Misuse of Drugs Regulations (2001) define the classes of person authorized to supply and possess controlled drugs.
➤ Controlled drugs are normally stored in a locked cupboard within a locked cupboard.
➤ There is a special procedure in giving a controlled drug.
➤ Only the nurse in charge of the ward can order a controlled drug.
➤ Controlled drugs are ordered and catalogued in separate books and registers.

→

Supply and administration of medicines

➢ Nurses can now be involved in the supply and administration of medicines.
➢ The *Supply and Administration of Medicines Under Group Protocols Report* lays down specific criteria which must be adhered to.

Prescribing law and non-medical prescribing

➢ Nurses and pharmacists can now prescribe medicines and medicinal products.
➢ Nurses can now be supplementary prescribers provided they follow agreed clinical management plans.
➢ Changes that took place in 2006 enabled nurses and pharmacists to take a further step and prescribe independently to an agreed clinical management plan.

Multiple choice questions

Try answering these multiple choice questions to test what you have learned from reading this chapter. You can check your answers on page 203.

1 The Misuse of Drugs Act was published in which year?

a) 1975
b) 1971
c) 1970
d) 2001

2 Which class of drug is morphine?

a) A
b) B
c) C
d) D

3 Which schedule does cannabis belong to?

a) 5
b) 3
c) 2
d) 1

←

4 What does PGD stand for?

a) Patient Group Direction
b) Prescribing Good Drugs
c) Public Grouped Decisions
d) Patient Generated Directions

5 Most drugs have two names. What are they?

a) General and specific
b) Pharmacological and popular
c) Generic and brand
d) Hospital and manufacturers

6 If you gave a drug covertly to a capable adult in law you would have committed what?

a) A slander
b) A defamation
c) A trespass
d) A Libel

7 If an adult lacks the capacity to consent, can another person consent on their behalf?

a) Yes
b) No
c) Only in an emergency
d) Only under a CMP

8 Which of the following allied health professionals cannot prescribe?

a) Occupational therapist
b) Pharmacist
c) Nurse
d) Physiotherapist

9 What is the most important factor in facilitating the reporting of drug errors?

a) Reading the NMC's guidelines
b) Weekly drug audit meetings
c) A robust drugs policy
d) A no-blame culture

←

10 Tampering or crushing of a medicine is unlawful because

a) It effects the pharmacokinetics and dynamics
b) It invalidates the product licence
c) It means that you cannot predict the side-effects
d) It does not involve a pharmacist

For further assistance with calculations, please see Meriel Hutton's *Essential Calculation Skills for Nurses, Midwives and Healthcare Practitioners* (Open University Press 2009).

Recommended further reading

Beckwith, S. and Franklin, P. (2007) *Oxford Handbook of Nurse Prescribing*. Oxford: Oxford University Press.

Brenner, G.M. and Stevens, C.W. (2006) *Pharmacology*, 2nd edn. Philadelphia, PA: Saunders Elsevier.

Clayton, B.D. (2009) *Basic Pharmacology for Nurses*, 15th edn. St Louis, MO: Mosby Elsevier.

Coben, D. and Atere-Roberts, E. (2005) *Calculations for Nursing and Healthcare*, 2nd edn. Basingstoke: Palgrave Macmillan.

DH (Department of Health) (1989) *Report of the Advisory Group on Nurse Prescribing* (Crown Report). London: DoH.

DH (Department of Health) (1998) *Review of Prescribing, Supply and Administration of Medicines: A Report on the Supply and Administration of Medicines Under Group Protocols*. London: DH.

DH (Department of Health) (1999) *A Review of Prescribing, Supply and Administration of Medicines – Final Report* (Crown Report 2). London: DH.

DH (Department of Health) (2000) *NHS Plan: A Plan for Investment, a Plan for Reform*. London: DH.

DH (Department of Health) (2005) *Supplementary Prescribing by Nurses, Pharmacists, Chiropodists/Podiatrists, Physiotherapists and Radiographers within the NHS in England: a Guide for Implementation*. London: DH.

DHSS (Department of Health and Social Security) (1986) *Neighbourhood Nursing: A Focus for Care* (Cumberlege Report). London: HMSO.

Downie, G., Mackenzie, J. and Williams, A. (2007) *Pharmacology and Medicines Management for Nurses*, 4th edn. Edinburgh: Churchill Livingstone.

Gatford, J.D. and Phillips, N. (2006) *Nursing Calculations*, 7th edn. Edinburgh: Churchill Livingstone Elsevier.

Karch, A.M. (2008) *Focus on Nursing Pharmacology*, 4th edn. Philadelphia, PA: Lippincott Williams & Wilkins.

Lapham, R. and Agar, H. (2003) *Drug Calculations for Nurses: A Step-by-step Approach*, 2nd edn. London: Arnold.

NHS UK (2005) Managing someone's legal affairs, www.nhs.uk/CarersDirect/moneyandlegal/legal/Pages/MentalCapacityAct.aspx.

NMC (Nursing and Midwifery Council) (2008) *Standards for Medicines Management*. London: NMC.

NMC (Nursing and Midwifery Council) (2008) *Code of Professional Conduct*. London: NMC.

Simonson, T., Aarbakke, J., Kay, I., Coleman, I., Sinnott, P. and Lyssa, R. (2006) *Illustrated Pharmacology for Nurses*. London: Hodder Arnold.

Trounce, J. (2000) *Clinical Pharmacology for Nurses*, 16th edn. New York: Churchill Livingstone.

Conclusion

In order to become safe in the administration of medicines and become competent in the education of patients with regard to their medication, the nurse must have knowledge of basic pharmacology and physiology. Also, in the interests of patient safety, they must be able to complete simple drug calculations. This book has introduced you to the knowledge necessary when engaging in these skills.

The focus of your career is nursing and it is important that any science subject is applied to that discipline. The clinical tips have been designed to give you an insight into the importance of understanding pharmacology and to be relevant to the process of nursing. We hope that the first two chapters managed to set the scene in terms of introducing topics and concepts that enabled you to understand Chapters 3 to 8 in more depth.

Chapters 3 to 8 should have given you a feel for the fascinating world of pharmacology and also demonstrated to you how important this concept is to nursing. The links to physiology should have been helpful in terms of your understanding. We hope that the breadth and depth of the discussion has left you wanting to read further and there are many books out there which can give you more detail and cover a wider range of medicines.

Chapter 9 should have given you an insight into the patient's role and responsibility with regard to their medicine management. Nurses generally are well placed to help patients understand the need to adhere to instruction and advice. Often the nurse is the agent of continuity in the patient's journey, therefore we hope you have gained some insight into the importance of your role as a health educator.

Several studies during the past few years have suggested that nurses were not very accurate in drug calculations. This resulted in changes taking place at a pre-registration education level. Most universities now test the competence of their students in drug calculations by either formal or informal methods. We hope that the questions at the end of most chapters were realistic and helped you to practise your mathematics in relation to drug dosages.

The whole area of giving a medicine is fraught with potential pitfalls. That is why we hope you enjoyed Chapter 10. Calculating the correct dose is obviously important, but there remain other areas of law and professional standards which need upholding if you are to become a safe practitioner.

Overall we hope this book has given you the motivation and interest to want to increase your knowledge in this important area of nursing. There are many texts that you can refer to as you become more knowledgeable and inquisitive (see our suggestions for further reading). We hope that our book has been one of the first stepping stones in your chosen career as a nurse.

Glossary

A

absorption: process by which a drug reaches the general circulation and becomes biologically available.

acetylcholine: chemical transmitter released by certain nerve endings.

adrenaline: hormone produced by adrenal medulla to prepare the body for fight or flight.

antidote: a remedy which counteracts the action of a chemical.

anti-emetic: a drug given to stop nausea and vomiting.

aperient: a drug given to help loosen the bowels.

arachidonic acid: substance liberated from the cell enabling the cyclo-oxygenase pathway.

B

basophil: a granular white cell which contains heparin and histamine.

bioavailability: the extent and rate of a drug that becomes available to its target receptor following administration.

blood-brain barrier (BBB): the membranes between the circulating blood and the brain.

b-lymphycyte: a type of white cell associated with the immune response and production of antibodies.

bradykinin: powerful pain-producing substance.

C

chemotaxis: the movement of white cells towards an area of inflammation.

collagen: an essential protein that helps make up many tissues in the body.

complement proteins: a group of proteins which are essential in aiding the inflammatory response.

cyclo-oxygenase pathway: a metabolic pathway which results in the formation of prostoglandins.

cytochrome P450: a group of enzymes which help metabolize drugs.

D

decongestant: a drug used to unblock the upper respiratory tract.

distribution: the distribution of drugs after absorption, to reach their target sites.

dopamine: neurotransmitter implicated in movement.

E

elimination: removal of drugs and their metabolites from the body.

enteric coating: protective coating which ensures a medicine is released after leaving the stomach.

extrinsic pathway: blood clotting mechanism which is initiated by external damage to vessel.

F

first pass: effect caused by metabolism of a drug by the liver resulting in only part of the drug reaching the circulation.

G

gamma-aminobutyric acid (GABA): neurotransmitter associated with a dampening effect on brain activity.

glucocorticoid: hormones secreted by the adrenal cortex.

H

half life: time taken for a drug to lose 50 per cent of its plasma concentration in the body.

histamine: substance which causes widespread vasodilation and increased permeability of blood vessels.

I

ingestion: taking into the body.

intramuscular (IM): injection into a muscle.

intravenous (IV): injection directly into a vein.

intrinsic pathway: blood clotting mechanism initiated without any external damage needed to vessel.

L

laxative: drug given to promote defecation.

M

mycobacteria: rod-shaped acid fast bacteria implicated in tuberculosis.

N

neuroleptics: antipsychotic drugs.

P

phantom limb pain: the sensation of pain that is still reported from a patient after the removal of a limb/body part.

plasma protein: proteins carried in the plasma with a range of physiological functions. Target sites for drug binding.

plasminogen: inactive plasma protein.

potassium: major intracellular cation.

prostacyclin: prostaglandin implicated in making platelets less sticky.

proteolytic enzymes: enzymes which break down proteins within the cell membrane.

prothrombin: inactive plasma protein involved in blood clotting.

proton pump inhibitor (PPI): drug which stops production of hydrochloric acid in the stomach.

R

renin: a hormone secreted by the kidney to help raise blood pressure.

S

salicylates: group of drugs including aspirin which are acidic and given as analgesics.

septicaemia: overwhelming infection of the blood.

serotonin: neurotransmitter implicated in alterations of mood.

steady state: this is the point reached when the amount of drug being absorbed is the same as the amount being excreted.

subcutaneous (SC): injection given into tissue just beneath the skin.

T

therapeutic range: the range of plasma drug concentration in which medicine has its best effect.

therapeutic index: this is the comparison of the amount of a drug needed to bring about a therapeutic response to the amount that would cause a toxic effect.

thromboxane: implicated in making platelets more sticky.

topically: the application of a drug directly to skin and mucous membranes.

Answers

Chapter 1

Case study ①, Mrs Asamoah

The following areas of assessment would help you identify factors influencing the absorption and distribution of the medication which Mrs Asamoah is taking.

- Assess Mrs Asamoah's mobility
- Assess the drug formulation: does she require liquids instead of tablets?
- Assess her age in relationship to plasma protein loss
- Assess if she is dehydrated
- Assess her nutritional status and when she takes her medicines in relationship to meals
- Is she taking any OTC medication?
- Check the BNF for any interactions between drugs that may affect absorption and distribution

Case study ②, Mr Mambety

The following factors may influence Mr Mambety's ability to metabolise and excrete drugs during his post-operative recovery.

- Think of alcohol effects on liver
- Think about the effects of smoking on the systems of the body
- Consider the effects of surgery on the movement of the intestine
- Check the fluid balance
- Check the urinary output

Calculations

1   2000mcg
2   0.6g
3   1200mg
4   1g in 10,000 is the weakest
5   360ml
6   2 tablets
7   2 tablets

Multiple choice questions

1   A
2   A
3   D
4   C
5   B
6   B
7   D
8   B
9   D
10 A

Chapter 2

Case study ①, Marek Brodzki

Your responsibilities regarding the antibiotics are:

- This may be a mild allergy
- Needs to be closely monitored
- No treatment necessary, although may give antihistamines
- Report rash to doctor
- The rash may become a more severe reaction

Your responsibilities regarding recording the incident are:

- Record extent of the rash, when first noticed: is it becoming worse, how irritant is it?
- Marek to tell health care professionals of any suggestion of antibiotic reaction

Your responsibilities regarding prevention of a re-occurance are:

- Marek should inform health care staff if other members of the family have reactions
- Ensure it is documented on the patient's prescription chart and notes if he has an allergy
- Marek to carry information with him if he suspects a severe reaction (e.g. bracelet or medical card)

Case study ②, Sue Kent

According to the BNF:

- Ibuprofen increases the actions of warfarin
- Sue may take some drugs like a COX2 inhibitor

Multiple choice questions

1	B
2	C
3	B
4	D
5	A
6	C
7	C
8	D
9	B
10	A

Chapter 3

Case study ①, Dawn Mason

The mode of action:

- Actions on prostaglandins and nociceptors
- Talk about the cyclo-oxygenase pathway
- Opiates block calcium channels in pain pathways
- Opiates open potassium channels
- Opiates bind with receptors

The importance of stepping down from opiates to NSAIDS would involve:

- Give NSAIDs before taking Dawn off opiates
- Discuss analgesic ladder

The maintenance required to achieve a steady plasma concentration would involve:

- Make sure Dawn is taking regular doses so a steady state is achieved
- Ensure you evaluate Dawn's level of pain so that you know a steady level of analgesia has been maintained
- Discuss side-effects

You would explain the information by:

- Using understandable terms, diagrams or models and check the health care assistant's understanding

Case study ②, Alex Smith

Mode of action of paracetamol and NSAIDS would involve:

- Actions of the drugs on cyclo-oxygenase pathway 2 (COX2) and cyclo-oxygenase pathway 3 (COX3)

The need for regulator dosing to achieve therapeutic plasma concentrations would involve:

- Ensuring you evaluate Alex's level of pain so that you know a steady level of analgesia has been maintained
- Making sure Alex is taking regular doses so a steady state is achieved
- Discussing side-effects

You would explain the information by:

- Checking Alex's and his parents' knowledge, plan information session, writing and agreeing learning outcomes, using understandable terms, using diagrams or models and checking their understanding.

Calculations

1   1.5ml
2   50ml
3   3 tablets: 20mg + 20mg + 10mg
4   2.6ml
5   0.8ml
6   1.5ml
7   8 tablets
8   0.4ml
9   0.7ml
10   0.75ml

Multiple choice questions

1   A
2   D
3   B
4   D
5   C
6   B
7   A
8   C
9   D
10   C

Chapter 4

Case study ①, Cynthia Day

Clarithromycin is:

- Bacteriostatic at low levels
- Bacteriocidal at high levels
- Inhibits protein synthesis
- Prescribed in penicillin allergy

The possible reasons why this drug has been chosen are:

- Active against most gram positive bacteria
- Active against many penicillin resistant bacteria
- Useful in treating respiratory tract infections
- Safe and least toxic of antibiotics

The clinical observations which would need conducting on Mrs Day are:

- Trend of pyrexia
- Cardiovascular status
- Nutritional and fluid status – promoting absorption, distribution and elimination of the drug
- Respiratory function and sputum examination (effect of drug)
- GI disturbances – side-effects of drug
- Skin rashes and pruritus – side-effects of drug

Case study ②, Ella Jackson

The discussion on the difference between bacteria and viruses may include:

- Types of bacteria
- Difference between gram negative and gram positive
- Difference between our cells and bacterial cells

Mechanism of actions of antibiotics would include:

- Discussing how antibiotics work in different ways to destroy bacteria
- The difference between a bacteria and a virus

Alternative medications to relieve Ella's symptoms may include:

- Discussing use of pain relief and antipyretics

Calculations

1   16ml
2   1.7ml
3   40ml
4   2 tablets
5   4.5ml
6   56 tablets
7   10ml
8   2ml
9   7.5ml
10   20ml

Multiple choice questions

1 C
2 A
3 C
4 B
5 D
6 D
7 A
8 C
9 C
10 D

Chapter 5

Case study ①, Radu Beligan

Action of steroids on the body may include:

- Steroids affect COX2 pathway

Discussion of the side effects of steroids may include:

- Increases blood glucose
- Less protein production
- Affects fat distribution in the body
- Sodium is retained
- Calcium is removed from bone
- Secondary diabetes
- Secondary hypertension
- Low blood calcium
- Lowered wound healing
- Lowered ability to fight infection

Other information that may be given to Mr Beligan may include:

- Need to carry card
- Do not suddenly stop taking medication
- Keep good stock of drug
- Inform the doctor and dentist

Case study ②, Louise Mason

Discussion on the mode of action of ibuprofen, steroids and methotrexate may include:

- Discussion about prostaglandin synthesis
- Discussion about COX2 pathway

- Discussion about arachidonic acid formation
- Discussion about DNA in a cell and how methotrexate works on this

Discussion regarding maintaining drug therapy between stopping one drug and commencing another could include:

- Explaining steroids are only needed until the methotrexate begins to work

Discussion of the possible side-effects of steroids may include:

- Explaining the side-effects of steroids including high blood pressure, secondary diabetes, poor wound healing, masking of infection
- Checking Louise's parents' knowledge, plan session, writing/agreeing learning outcomes, using understandable terms, using diagrams or models and check their understanding

Calculations

1 6 tablets
2 5 tablets
3 The nearest accurate dose would be 3.4ml
4 3ml
5 The nearest accurate dose would be 4.3ml
6 2 tablets
7 600mg in each dose
8 The nearest accurate dose is 0.75ml
9 3.2ml
10 0.5ml

Multiple choice questions

1 D
2 A
3 C
4 A
5 B
6 C
7 D
8 C
9 B
10 A

Chapter 6

Case study, Olek Krupa

The advice that you would give Mr Krupa with regard to taking warfarin may include:

- Importance of carrying an anticoagulant card highlighting dosage
- Essential to make and keep blood check appointment
- To inform any doctor, nurse or dentist that he is receiving anticoagulant therapy
- To take tablets as prescribed
- To avoid alcohol, drugs containing aspirin and any other OTC medications
- To make an appointment with the GP or anticoagulant clinic if he notices any bleeding, bruising or indigestion
- To adjust lifestyle to avoid unnecessary trauma – for example, to be careful when using sharp gardening or domestic implements

Calculations

1 5ml
2 4 tablets
3 0.525ml
4 0.9ml
5 3 tablets
   5mg + 1mg + 1mg = 7mg
   or
   1mg + 3mg + 3mg = 7mg
6 5ml per hour
7 0.1ml
8 500 units 6 40ml = 20,000 units
   20,000 units 7 5000 units = 4ml
   4ml of heparin and 36ml of saline = 40ml of solution
9 0.9ml
10 a) 0.25ml
   b) 0.25ml
   c) 0.5ml

Multiple choice questions

1 C
2 A
3 A
4 D
5 C
6 B
7 A
8 C
9 C
10 D

Chapter 7

Case study ①, Joseph Olita

Discussion with reference to action of corticosteroid and bronchodilator may include:

- Reference to bronchodilators
- Reference to adrenoreceptors and stimulation of such receptors
- Reference to steroids and arachidonic acid
- Mention local side-effects like sore or dry throat
- Mention possibility of thrush formation

Discussion on inhaler technique may involve:

- Talking Joseph through the inhaler technique outlined earlier in the chapter

You would explain the information by:

- Checking his knowledge, planning the session, writing/agreeing learning outcomes, using understandable terms, using diagrams/models

Case study ②, Elizabeth Jones

Discussion with reference to the action of corticosteroid salbutamol on the airways may include:

- Reference to bronchodilators
- Reference to adrenoreceptors and stimulation of such receptors
- Reference to steroids and arachidonic acid
- Mention local side-effects like sore or dry throat
- Mention of possibility of thrush formation

Discussion to assuage Elizabeth's concerns may include:

- Checking her knowledge, planning the session, writing/agreeing learning outcomes, using understandable terms, using diagrams/models

Calculations

1	2ml
2	8ml
3	3 tablets
4	2ml
5	1.25ml
6	0.5ml
7	2ml
8	12.5ml
9	0.28ml
10	45ml

Multiple choice questions

1	B
2	D
3	A
4	C
5	C
6	B
7	D
8	B
9	A
10	C

Chapter 8

Case study ①, Debbie Butcher

How SSRIs work would be explained by:

- Checking Debbie's knowledge, planning the session, using understandable terms, using diagrams/models and checking her understanding of what you have told her
- Discussing the monoamine theory of depression
- Discussing what serotonin is and what is implicated with regard to mood
- Explaining what happens normally at a synapse
- Explaining how SSRIs affect the re-uptake of serotonin

Case study ②, Anil Kahn

You would discuss the action of atypical drugs including the following:

- Drugs block the dopaminergic pathways in the brain
- Most typical antipsychotic medication acts on D_2 receptors
- Most atypical antipsychotic medication acts on D_1 and D_4 receptors

Discussion regarding the difference between atypical and typical antipsychotics could include:

- Typical drugs are associated with more side-effects
- Atypical drugs are better at dealing with negative symptoms of schizophrenia
- Patients often gain weight and suffer secondary diabetes from atypical drugs

Calculations

1	2 tablets
2	3 tablets
3	4 tablets
4	2.5 tablets
5	0.4ml
6	0.25ml
7	2.5ml
8	1ml
9	4ml
10	2.5ml

Multiple choice questions

1	D
2	C
3	D
4	A
5	D
6	B

7   A
8   C
9   B
10   C

Chapter 9

Case study ①, Kubi Garise

Strategies to compare Mrs Garise's compliance may include:

- Linking medication-taking with brushing teeth in the morning and evening
- Taking medications at coffee or tea breaks
- Taking medications at the same time as a favourite programme
- Involving others in ensuring medicines are being taken
- Placing notes or reminders around the house
- Wearing an alarm watch that goes off when tablets are due
- Keeping a diary of when tablets have been taken
- Discussing pill organizing box

Case study ②, Ella Jenkins

Discussion regarding the importance of compliance with the patient may include:

- Checking the mother's knowledge, planning the session, using understandable terms, using diagrams/models and checking her understanding
- Ascertaining if Mrs Jenkins appreciates the importance of Ella taking her medicine
- Ascertaining if Mrs Jenkins understands the consequences of Ella *not* taking her medicine

Improving the patient compliance with taking the antibiotics may be improved by:

- Considering looking at the formulation. Can the drug be given as a syrup which has a flavour Ella will like?

Calculations

1   2 tablets
2   2500g
3   0.12ml
4   1,250,000mcg
5   2.5ml
6   2.5ml
7   200ml per hour
8   100,000mg
9   25g
10   300g

Multiple choice questions

1   A
2   C
3   B
4   D
5   B
6   A
7   D
8   C
9   D
10   B

Chapter 10

Case study ①, Mr Ajani

- The *patient medicines administration chart* is not a prescription but a direction to administer medication. It must be signed by a registered prescriber and authorizes the delegation to administer medication on the prescriber's behalf.
- Standard 2: registrants (1st and 2nd level) must check any direction to administer a medicinal product.
- Check that the prescription chart is signed and dated by the authorized prescriber.
- In exceptional circumstances, where medication (*not* including controlled drugs) has been previously prescribed and the prescriber is unable to issue a new prescription, but where changes to the dose are considered necessary, information technology (such as fax, text message or email) may be used but must confirm any change to the original prescription.

Case study ②, Mrs Simpson

Your answer to what conditions the nurse must have satisfied to become a prescriber and what are the advantages to Mrs Simpson of having a nurse prescriber could have included the following:

The nurse must have completed and passed an accredited non-medical prescribing course to gain notation on her NMC registration as a V300 prescriber. The fact the nurse is a prescriber and can issue the prescription provides Mrs Simpson with quicker access to medication. This allows for service improvement and greater patient satisfaction and can promote improved patient–professional relationships. Even though Mrs Simpson could, in theory, buy paracetamol over the counter, you should bear the following in mind:

- Her ability to go shopping.
- The limited number of tablets she would be able to buy in a pharmacy.
- The fact that Mrs Simpson is eligible for free prescriptions.

Multiple choice questions

1	B
2	A
3	D
4	A
5	C
6	C
7	D
8	A
9	D
10	B

Index

5-hydroxytryptamine 149, 153–6
P450 70

ABCDE approach 22
abciximab 108
absent seizures 136
absorption 4–6, 18, 23
   and ADR 18
   age-related ADR 23
   definition 13
acarbose 128
ACE inhibitors *see* angiotensin-converting enzyme
   inhibitors
acetylcholine antagonists 134–5
aching pain 33
aciclovir 66–7
acquired immuno-deficiency syndrome 55, 64–6, 68
   see also human immunodeficiency virus
action potential 30
Actrapid 125, 142, 175
acute inflammation 84–5
acute inflammatory exudate 84
acute multi-system severe type I hypersensitivity allergic
   reaction 22
   see also anaphylaxis
addictive effects 19
ADE *see* adverse drug event
adherence 168–9, 174
adjuvant drugs 36, 46
ADME 4
administration 182–3, 186
   correct site and method 182
   covert 182–3
   histamines 90
ADR *see* adverse drug reactions
adrenaline 37–9
adrenoceptors 8
adverse drug event 19–20
   Type A: augmented 20
   Type B: bizarre 20
   see also adverse drug reactions
adverse drug reactions 17–27
   adverse reactions 19–20
   age-related adverse drug reactions 22–4
   clinical significance of drug interactions 20–1
   definition 25
   introduction 18

main drug groups involved in adverse drug reactions
   21
   mechanisms of drug interactions 18–19
   minimizing effects of adverse drug reactions 21–2
adverse effects: aspirin 89
afferent neurones *see* sensory neurones
affinity 9
age-related ADRs 22–4
   absorption 23
   definition 25
   distribution 24
   metabolism 24
aggression 138
agitation states 171
agonistic drug action 9–10, 14
agoraphobia 149
agranulocytosis 159
AIDS *see* acquired immuno-deficiency syndrome
akathisia 159
albumin 18
alcohol 74, 150–1, 154, 156
alpha-adrenoreceptor antagonists 132
alpha-glucosidase inhibitors 128
alteplase 109, 111
alteration of medicines 184
amantadine 67
amenorrhea 159–60
amethocaine 36–7
amides 36–7
aminoglycosides 59
amitriptyline 153–4, 163
amobarbital 149
amoebic dysentery 74
amoeboflagellates 74
amoxacillin 57–8, 61, 78, 175
amphetamines 153
amphotericin 69
ampicillin 57
anaemia 45, 56
analgesia 44
analgesic ladder 39–40, *40*
analgesic mixture 46
analgesics 29–51
   analgesic ladder 39–40
   introduction 30–4
   local anaesthetics 36–9
   non-steroidal anti-inflammatory drugs 40–2

analgesics (*Continued*)
  opioid analgesics 42–6
  opioid antagonists 46–7
  paracetamol 42–3
  types of pain 34–6
anaphylactic shock 57
anaphylaxis 20, 22, 121
ancillary symptoms of depression 152
angiogenesis 85
angiotensin-converting enzyme inhibitors 19,
  130–2
anhedonia 152, 155, 157
anions 30
ankylosing spondylitis 87
anorexia 92–3, 127, 137
antagonistic drug action 9–10, 14
anti-inflammatory drugs 83–99
  antirheumatoid drugs 91–4
  aspirin 88–9
  cyclo-oxygenase pathway 2 inhibitors 88
  histamine 89
  introduction 84–6
  non-steroidal anti-inflammatory drugs 86–8
  paracetamol 89
  steroids 89–91
antibiotic reaction 24
antibiotic resistance 61
anticholinergia 154, 160
anticoagulant therapy 101–14
  blood clotting and thrombosis 103
  drugs that act on clotting cascade 104–9
  introduction 102–3
anticonvulsants 35–6, 136
antidepressants 8, 151–4, **154**
  tricyclic 153–4
  types of **154**
antiemetics 46
antifungal drugs 69–72, **71**
  amphotericin 69
  azoles 70
  definition 77–8
  flucystosine 71
  future antifungal therapy 72
  griseofulvin 70
  nystatin 69–70
  terbinafine 72
antifungal therapy 72
antigens 85
antihistamines 46, 89, 96, 160
antihypertensive therapy 134
antimicrobials 53–81
  antibiotic resistance 61
  antifungal drugs 69–72
  beta-lactam antibiotics 56–8
  drugs to treat tuberculosis 62–3

fungal infections 68–9
human immunodeficiency virus 64–6
inhibition of bacterial DNA 60
interference with folate 55–6
interference with synthesis 58–60
introduction 54–5
issues with neonates and children 61–2
other antiviral drugs 66–8
protozoa 72–5
viral disease 63–4
antiobiotic resistance 61, 76
antiplatelet drugs 108
  abciximab 108
  aspirin 108
  clopidogrel 108
antipsychotics 151, 158–9
antipyretic drugs 40
antiretroviral therapy 65
antirheumatoid drugs 91–4
  chloroquine 93
  definition 96
  gold compounds 92
  leflunomide 93–4
  methotrexate 93
  penicillamine 92–3
  sulfasalazine 92
antithrombin III 103–6
antiviral drugs 66–8
  aciclovir 66–7
  amantadine 67
  definition 77
  ganciclovir 67
  immunoglobulins 67–8
  interferons 68
anxiety 148–52
  behavioural inhibition system 149
  classifications of 148
  defence system 148–9
  definition 161
  management of 149–52
  neurotransmitters in 149
anxiolytic treatment 149
apicomplexa 72–3
apprehension 148
arachidonic drugs 40, 86, 120
arthritis 91–4
ascending pain pathways *35*
aspergillus 68
aspirin 41, 88–9, 108, 112
  adverse effects of 89
  definition 95, 111
  overdose 89
asthma 116–21, 139
  in children 117–18
  definition 140

drugs used in treating 118–21
  management of 120–1, **121**
  pathological changes in 116–17
  risk factors 117
  well-controlled 139
ataxia 137
Atenolol 12
atherosclerosis 103, 128–9
athlete's foot 68
atrial fibrillation 24
attention deficit 157
atypical antipsychotics 159
augmented drug reaction 20
auranofin 92
autoimmunity 85
autonomic arousal 148
Avandia 128
avoidance behaviour 149
awareness of medication need 169
axons 30
azaspirodecanediones 151
azoles 70
  fluconazole 70
  ketoconazole 70
  miconazole 70

B-lymphocytes 116–17
bacteria types 54–5
bacterial DNA 60
bacterial infection 54–5
barbiturate binding *150*
barbiturates 149–50
basic drug calculation formula 11–12
basic receptor theory *10*
BBB *see* blood–brain barrier
beclometasone 90, 120–1, 140
behavioural inhibition system 149
Bendroflumethazide 19, 130, 142
benign hypertension 129–30
benzodiazepines 8, 21, 23, 45, 149–50,
  160
benzylpenicillin 56
beta$_2$ adrenoreceptor agonists 10, 118
beta blockers 19, 130–2, 139, 151, 160
beta-adrenergic blockers 150–1
beta-adrenoreceptor antagonists 131
  see also beta blockers
beta-lactam antibiotics 56–8
  cephalosporins 57
  clavulanic acid 57–8
  definition 75
  penicillins 56–7
beta-lactamase inhibitor 57–8
Biers block 38–9
Bifidobacterium bifidus 61

biological factors contributing to depression 153
  hormonal influences 153
  monoamine hypothesis 153
biotransformation 6–7
  definition 13
  hepatic metabolism 7
  see also metabolism
biphasic isophane insulin 125–6
bipolar depression 152, 156
bipolar disorder 130
bizarre drug reaction 20
blockbuster drugs 61
blood clotting 102–3
  constriction of blood vessel 102
  definition 110
  dissolving of fibrin clot 103
  formation of fibrin/blood clot 102–3
  formation of platelet plug 102
blood flow 4
blood vessel constriction 102
blood–brain barrier 6, 57, 59–60, 62–3, 68, 133
BNF *see* British National Formulary
body fluids 6
body's analgesic system 33–4
bovine spongiform encephalopathy 54
bradykinin 31, 33, 40
British National Formulary 9, 18, 20, 24, 150, 157, 181
bronchoconstriction 116–17, 119
bronchodilation 118–21
bronchospasm 121, 131
BSE *see* bovine spongiform encephalopathy
budesonide 120, 140
bupivacaine 36, 38
buprenorphine 185
buspirone 151

calcium antagonists 130, 132, 136–7
candida 61, 69–70
Candida albicans 69
Candida krusei 72
candidiasis 120
captopril 131
Carbamazepine 107, 142, 156–7
cardiac rhythm problems 154
cations 31
caudal anaesthesia 38
causes of antibiotic resistance 61
celecoxib 88, 95
cephalosporins 57
Certoparin 105
cerufoxamine 57
channel blockers 8, 36–7
channel modulators 8
chemical stability 5
chemotaxis 84

child abuse 152
children 61–2, 117–18
   asthma in 117–18
chloramphenicol 58–9, 109
chloroquine 93
chlorpromazine 134
Christmas disease 104
chronic conditions 115–45
   asthma 116–18
   chronic obstructive pulmonary disease 121–2
   diabetes 122–3
   drugs used to treat asthma 118–21
   epilepsy 135–9
   hypertension 128–32
   introduction 116
   medicine management of diabetes 123–8
   Parkinson's disease 132–5
chronic inflammation 85–6
chronic obstructive pulmonary disease 119, 121–2, 140
Cimetidine 107
ciprofloxacin 60
Citalopram 155, 160, 170
classifications of anxiety 148
clavulanic acid 57–8
Clexane 105
clindamycin 60
clinical management plan 187
clinical significance of drug interactions 20–1
   definition 25
   pharmacovigilance 21
   Type A ADR 20
   Type B ADR 20
   yellow card system 21
clopidogrel 108, 111
Clostridium difficile 60
clot blusters see fibrinolytic drugs
clotting cascade 104–9
clozapine 159
CMP see clinical management plan
co-codamol 12, 46
co-trimoxazole 55
cocaine 36, 45, 153
codeine 6–7, 40, 44–6, 185
coma 72–3, 89, 136
Committee on Safety of Medicines 58, 150
competence in consent 183–4
competing effects of drugs 19
competitive antagonists 10
compliance 168–9, 174
concept of affinity 9
concordance 168–9, 174
conduction anaesthesia 38
confusion 171
congestive heart failure 41–2

conjunctivitis 58, 64
consent 182–3
consequences of not taking medication 169–70
constipation 45, 160
constriction of blood vessel 102
contact time 4
contraindications 41, 57
controlled drugs 61, 185–6
COPD see chronic obstructive pulmonary disease
correct medicine 180–1
cortex/limbic system 158
corticosteroids 119–21, 139, 153
   inhaled 119–21
cough reflex depression 44
covert administration of medicine 182–3
critical incident analysis 184–5
cromoglicate 121
Crown, June 187
CSM see Committee on Safety of Medicines
Cumberlege, Julia 187
cyclo-oxygenase pathway 2 inhibitors 88
   celecoxib 88
   definition 95
cyclo-oxygenase pathways 42–3, 86, 86, 87
cytochrome P450 70, 119
cytomegalo virus 67

Dabigatran 107
Dalkeparin 105
Dangerous Drug Act 1967 185
death 117, 119
defence system 148–9
degree of ionization 5–6
dementia 173
dendrites 30
deoxyribonucleic acid 60, 63–5
Department of Health 18, 186–7
depolarization 31, 37
depression 138, 152–7
   ancillary symptoms 152
   biological factors 153
   definition 161–2
   genetic factors 153
   key symptoms 152
   management of 153–7
   psychological factors 152
development of thrombosis 103, 110
DH see Department of Health
diabetes mellitus 66, 122–8
   definition 140
   management of 123–8
   tablets used in **129**
   types of **124**
diabetic neuropathy 35

diamorphine 44
diarrhoea 57, 59–60, 62–3, 67, 73–4, 93–4, 127–8, 155
diazepam 150, 180
diclofenac 41–2
Digoxin 21, 23, 174
Dipyridamole 102
disease-modifying antirheumatoid drugs 91–4
dissolving fibrin clot 103
distribution 6, 18–19, 24
    and ADR 18–19
    age-related ADR 24
    definition 13
diuretics 19, 21, 23
dizziness 20, 42, 45, 60, 67, 73, 89, 92–3, 105, 137, 154
DMARDs see disease-modifying antirheumatoid drugs
DNA see deoxyribonucleic acid
dopamine receptor agonists 132–4, 154
doxazosin 132
drug action 8–9
    affinity 9
    definition 13–14
    first pass metabolism 9
drug binding 8
drug error reporting 184–5
drug interactions 17–27
    see also adverse drug reactions
drug specificity 10
drugs that act on clotting cascade 104–9
    antiplatelet drugs 108
    enoxaparin 105
    fibrinolytic drugs 108–9
    future anticoagulant therapy 107
    heparin 104–5
    hirudin 106
    low molecular weight heparins 105
    vitamin K 104
    warfarin 106–7
drugs that treat asthma 118–21
    beta$_2$ adrenoreceptor agonists 118
    cromoglicate 121
    definition 140
    inhaled corticosteroids 119–21
    ipratropium 119
    methylxanthines 119
    muscarinic receptor antagonists 119
drugs to treat tuberculosis 62–3, 76
dynorphins 34
dysentery 72, 74
dysesthesia 35
dyskinesia 134
dyspepsia 41
dyspnoea 116, 118, 121
dysrhythmias 73, 119
dystonia 159

ear infection 61, 75, 173
    and compliance 173
efferent neurones see motor neurones
EMLA cream 37
empowerment in chronic disease management 171–4
    patient education 171–2
    patient as partner in decision-making 172–3
Enalopril 8
endocytosis 64
endorphins 34
enhancement of GABA action 137–8
    sodium valproate 137–8
    vigabatrin 138
enkephalins 34
enoxaparin 105, 110
Entamoeba histolytica 74
Enterococcus faecalis 61
enterohepatic recirculation 7
enzyme inducers 19, 137
enzyme inhibitors 19
enzymes 8
eosinophils 117
epidural anaesthesia 38
epilepsy 135–9
    definition 141
    drugs used in **139**
    enhancement of GABA action 137–8
    generalized seizures 136
    inhibition of calcium functions 137
    inhibition of sodium channel function 136–7
    partial seizures 135–6
equivalencies of weight **11**
erythromycin 59–60, 78
esmachs bandage 38–9
ester agents 36
ethosuximide 137
eucosanoids 86
eukaryotes 55
euphoria 44
excretion 7, 19, 24
    and ADR 19
    age-related ADR 24
    definition 13
exsanguination 38–9
extradural anaesthesia 38
extrinsic pathway 102–3

factor III 102
factor IX 104, 106
factor VIII 102, 104
factors influencing effective medicine use 169–71, 174
    ability to obtain prescription 170–1
    confusion/agitation states 171
    consequences of not taking medicine 169

factors influencing effective medicine use (*Continued*)
    interaction with other medication 170
    patient awareness of medication need 169
    product formulation 170
    product packaging 170
    side-effects 170
    time of dosing 170
'fear, flight, fight' mechanism 148–9
fentanyl 44–5
fibrin formation 102–3
fibrinolytic drugs 108–9
    alteplase 109
    streptokinase 109
firing of neurone *32*
first pass metabolism 9
flagellates 73–4
flattened affect 157, 162
flatulence 128
flucloxacillin 57
fluconazole 70, 72
flucystosine 71
fluoroquinolones 60
fluoxetine 8, 151, 155, 160
flupentixol 151, 156, 158, 161, 163
folate 55–6
formation of fibrin 102–3
formation of platelet plug 102
free drugs 6
frusimide 130
fungal infections 68–9
    definition 77
    moulds 68
    true yeasts 68
    yeast-like fungi 69
future anticoagulant therapy 107, 111
future antifungal therapy 72

G-protein coupled receptors 8
GABA *see* gamma-aminobutyric acid
gabapentin 137
galactorrhoea 159–60
gamma-aminobutyric acid 136–7, 149–50
ganciclovir 67
gastrointestinal tract 18, 43–5
gate-controlled entry 33–4
generalized seizures 136
genetic factors contributing to depression 153
gentamycin 41, 59, 87–8, 175
GI *see* gastrointestinal tract
glaucoma 134
glipizide 127
glitazones 128
glucocorticoids 89–90, 119–20
gluconeogenesis 90
glyceryl trinitrate 9

gold compounds 92
gram stain 55
grand mal seizures 136
grey baby syndrome 59
griseofulvin 70
GTN *see* glyceryl trinitrate
gynaecomastia 159

H-receptors 89
Haemolytic streptococci 109
haemophilia 41, 104
haemorrhage 104, 108–9
haemostasis 102
half life 43, 65, 108–9, 127
hallucinations 67, 134–5, 157
haloperidol 151, 161, 163
healing by repair 85
health belief model 172
Health and Social Care Act 2001 187
heparin 104–5, 110, 112
hepatic metabolism 7
hepatitis 70
hepatoxicity 138
heroin 45
high blood pressure 109
Hippocrates 41
hirudin 106
histamine 33, 84, 89, 117, 121
    antihistamines 89
    definition 96
HIV *see* human immunodeficiency virus
HIV life cycle *66*
homeostasis 33, 40, 84, 102
hormonal influences of depression 153
hostility 138
human immunodeficiency virus 45, 64–6
    antiretroviral therapy 65
    definition 76
    non-nucleoside reverse transcriptase inhibitors 65
    nucleoside reverse transcriptase inhibitors 65
    protease inhibitors 65–6
Human Rights Act 1998 182
Hutton, Meriel 14, 49, 78, 97, 112, 142
hydrocortisone 71, 90, 97, 109
hyperglycaemia 90
Hypericum perforatum see St John's wort
hyperlipidaemia 66, 123
hyperplasia 137
hyperpolarization 44
hyperprolactinaemia 159
hypersensitivity 57, 137
hypertension 123, 128–33, 173
    alpha-adrenoreceptor antagonists 132
    angiotensin-converting enzyme inhibitors 131–2
    beta-adrenoreceptor antagonists 131

calcium antagonists 132
definition 141
drugs used in **133**
thiazide diuretics 130–1
hyperthermia 89
hypoglycaemia 126–7, 131, 151
hyponatraemia 70
hypoplasia 58
hypotension 73, 132, 154, 160

ibuprofen 40–2, 94, 97
identifying patient 180
IM action *see* intramuscular routes
immunoglobulin E 117
immunoglobulins 67–8
immunosuppression 61, 68–9
impotence 61
indigestion 119
inert drugs 6
infection 54
infectious disease 54–5
bacterial infection 54–5
see also antimicrobials
infertility 159–60
infiltration anaesthesia 38
inflammation 84–6
acute 84–5
chronic 85–6
inflammatory response *85*
inhaled corticosteroids 119–21
inhibition of bacterial DNA 60, 76
definition 76
fluoroquinolones 60
inhibition of calcium channels 137
ethosuximide 137
inhibition of sodium channel function 136–7
INR *see* international normalized ratio
insomnia 67
insulin 123–7
intermediate insulins 125
long-acting insulins 126
pumps 126–7
short-acting insulins 125
side-effects of 126
treatment with 123–5
types of **126**
insulin pumps 126–7
interaction with other medication 170
interference with folate 55–6
definition 75
trimethoprim 55–6
interference with protein synthesis 58–60
aminoglycosides 59
chloramphenicol 58–9
definition 75–6

lincosamides 60
macrolides 59
tetracyclines 58
interferons 68
intermediate insulins 125
international normalized ratio 42, 106–7
intestinal flora 58
intolerable side-effects 170
intramuscular routes 9
intravenous local anaesthesia 38–9
intravenous routes 9
intrinsic pathway 102–3
introduction to units/conversions 10–12, *11*
basic formula 11–12
inverse agonists 10
ion channels 8
ipratropium 119
ischaemia 108
Islets of Langerhans 122
isoniazid 62–3
isophane insulin 125
issues with neonates and children 61–2, 76
IV action *see* intravenous routes

Jacksonian seizure 136
jaundice 63
juvenile chronic arthritis 94
juvenile diabetes *see* diabetes mellitus

keratin 70
ketoconazole 70–1, 107
key symptoms of depression 152
kinase-linked receptors 8

Lactobacillus acidophilus 61
laxatives 46
leflunomide 93–4
legal and professional issues 179–92
alteration of medicines 184
controlled drugs 185–6
correct dose 181–2
correct medicine 180–1
correct patient 180
correct site and administration method 182
covert administration of medicines 182–3
introduction 180
mental capacity and competence in consent 183–4
prescribing law, non-medical prescribing 186–8
reporting drug errors 184–5
supply and administration of drugs 186
lethargy 62, 137
leucopenia 92
levodopa 133–4
life support principles 22
lifestyle conditions 116

ligand-gated ion channels 8
ligands 8
lignocaine 36–8
lincosamides 60
lipid to water coefficient 5
Lisinopril 19, 132
lithium 156–7
local anaesthetics 36–40, **40**
    definition 47–8
    extradural/epidural/caudal anaesthesia 38
    infiltration anaesthesia 38
    intravenous local anaesthesia 38–9
    mode of action 27
    nerve blockade 38
    preparation of 37
    spinal anaesthesia 38
    topical anaesthesia 37
    unwanted effects of 39
    see also analgesics
locus of control 173
long-acting insulins 126
low molecular weight heparins 105
low self-esteem 152
lysosomes 59
lysozome 84

macrolides 59
macrovascular disease 123
major drug groups in ADRs 21
malaria 72–3, 93
malignant hypertension 130
management of anxiety 149–52
    antidepressants 151–2
    antipsychotics 151
    azaspirodecanediones 151
    barbiturates 149–50
    benzodiazepines 150
    beta-adrenergic blockers 150–1
management of asthma 120–1
management of depression 153–7
    monoamine oxidase inhibitors 154
    other drugs 156–7
    St John's wort 157
    selective serotonin re-uptake inhibitors 154–6
    tricyclic antidepressants 153–4
management of diabetes 123–8
    insulin 123–7
    oral hypoglycaemic agents 127–8
MAOIs see monoamine ozidase inhibitors
mast cells 84, 117, 121
maturity onset diabetes see diabetes mellitus
mechanisms of drug interactions 18–19
    absorption 18
    definition 24–5
    distribution 18–19

excretion 19
metabolism 19
mechanisms of viruses 64
medicinal leeches 106
Medicinal Products: Prescription by Nurses Act 1992
    187
medicine management
    anxiety 149–52
    asthma 120–1
    depression 153–7
    diabetes 123–8
Medicines & Healthcare Products Regulatory Agency
    20–1
meglinitides 128
melaena 42, 105
Melzack, R. 33
memory impairment 171
meningitis 59, 68
mental capacity 183–4
Mental Capacity Act 2005 183
mental health 147–65
    anxiety 148–9
    depression 152–3
    introduction 148
    medicine management of anxiety 149–52
    medicine management of depression 153–7
    psychosis 157–60
meperidine 44
mesolimbic pathway 158–9
metabolism 6–7, **7**, 19, 24
    and ADR 19
    age-related ADR 24
metformin 127
methadone 44
methotrexate 93
methylxanthines 119
metronidazole 73–4
MHPRA see Medicines & Healthcare Products Regulatory
    Agency
miconazole 70–1
micro-orgasms 54
microvascular disease 123
minimizing effects of ADRs 21–2
    anaphylaxis 22
    treatment of anaphylaxis 22
mirtazapine 156
Misuse of Drugs Act 1971 185, 189
Misuse of Drugs Regulations 2001 185, **185**, 189
mixtard insulin 125
moclobemide 154
mode of action of local anaesthetics 37
molecular effects 8
    definition 13
    enzymes 8
    ion channels 8

receptors 8
   transport systems 8
monoamine hypothesis for depression 153
monoamine ozidase inhibitors 153–4
mood stabilization 156
morbidity 20, 162
morphine 34, 40, 44, 185
mortality 20
motor neurones 30
moulds 68
muscarinic receptor antagonists 119
myalgeia 68
mycelium 68
Mycobacterium tuberculosis 62
myelin 30, 33
myocardial infarction 9, 88, 129

n-acelylcysteine 43
NA *see* noradrenaline
Naloxone 45–6
naproxen 41, 87–8, 95
narrow therapeutic index 21
nateglinide 128
National Audit Office 168
National Institute for Health and Clinical Excellence 126, 156, 169
National Patient Safety Agency 180
nausea 44–5, 56, 59, 63, 67, 70, 73, 92–4, 127, 137, 155
nebulizers 118–19
Neighbourhood Nursing 187
neonates and children 19, 61–2
nephrotoxicity 59
nerve blockade 38
nerve impulse 30–1
nerve pain 34–6
neurokinin 31
neuroleptic malignant syndrome 160
neuroleptics 46
neurones 30, *31*
neuropathic pain 34–6
neurotransmitters 30, 149
   in anxiety 149
nevirapine 65
NHS Plan 187
NICE *see* National Institute for Health and Clinical Excellence
nigostriatal pathway 159
NMC *see* Nursing and Midwifery Council
nociceptive pain 34
nociceptors 31–3
non-adapting nociceptors 31
non-competitive antagonists 10
non-drug allergies 22
non-medical prescribing 186–8

non-nucleoside reverse transcriptase inhibitors 65, 77
non-steroid anti-inflammatory drugs 19, 40–2, 86–8
   aspirin 41
   definition 48, 95
   diclofenac 41–2
   ibuprofen 41
   naproxen 87–8
noradrenaline 149
normoglycaemia 123, 127
NPSA *see* National Patient Safety Agency
NRM *see* nucleus raphe magnus
NSAIDs *see* non-steroid anti-inflammatory drugs
nucleoside reverse transcriptase inhibitors 65, 77
nucleus raphe magnus 34
Nursing and Midwifery Council 180–1, 184, 188
   standards 188
nystagmus 137
nystatin 69–70

obesity 117
observation of patient 21
obsessive-compulsive disorder 148, 151–2
obtaining prescription 170–1
occupation 9–10
OCD *see* obsessive-compulsive disorder
Office for National Statistics 148
opiates 34
opioid analgesics 43–6
   codeine 45–6
   definition 48
   fentanyl 45
   morphine 44–5
opioid antagonists 46–7
   adjuvant drugs 46
optimal drug absorption 18
optimum drug performance 168
oral contraception 7, 63
oral hypoglycaemic agents 127–8
   alpha-glucosidase inhibitors 128
   mehlinitides 128
   metformin 127
   sulfonylureas 127–8
   thiazolidinediones 128
organ/tissue uptake 6
osteoarthritis 86, 91
osteoporosis 105
OTC medication *see* over the counter medication
other drugs to treat depression 156–7
ototoxicity 59
over the counter medication 22, 42–3, 58, 86, 181
overdosing 181–2
   on aspirin 89
   fentanyl 45
   on morphine 43

PABA *see* para-amino benzoic acid
PAG *see* periaqueductal grey
pain 30–6
   types of 34–6
pain reception 31–3
para-amino benzoic acid 36, 55
parabens 39
paracetamol 40, 42–3, 89
Parkinson's disease 132–5, 159
   acetylcholine antagonists 134–5
   definition 141
   dopamine receptor agonists 134
   drugs used in **135**
   levodopa 133–4
   selegiline 134
partial agonists 10
partial seizures 135–6
pathological changes in asthma 116–17
patient concordance 167–77
   adherence, compliance, concordance 168–9
   effective medicine use and concordance 169–71
   introduction 168
   patient empowerment in chronic disease
      management 171–3
patient education 171–2
patient group direction 186
patient as partner in decision-making 172–3
penicillamine 92–3
penicillins 56–7
peptidoglycan 56
periaqueductal grey 34
peripheral oedema 45
peritonitis 74
petit mal seizures 136
PGD *see* patient group direction
phagocites 59, 62
phantom limb pain 30
pharmacodynamics 3–16
   absorption 4–6
   agonistic and antagonistic drug action 9–10
   biotransformation 6–7
   distribution 6
   drug action 8–9
   drug specificity 10
   excretion 7
   general and molecular aspects 8
   introduction 4
   introduction to units/conversions 10–12
pharmacokinetics 3–16, **23**
   see also pharmacodynamics
pharmacovigilance 19–21
pharmakon 4, 21
phenalzine 154
phenobarbitone 142
phenytoin 136–7

photosensitivity 70, 92, 160
phytomenadiole 104, 106
pilocaine 36–9
pinpoint pupils 44
pioglitazone 128
plamsa protein binding 6
plasma clotting factors 102–3, **103**
plasminogen 103
Plasmodium falciparum 73
Plasmodium vivax 72
platelet plug formation 102
   antiplatelet drugs 108
polydypsia 123
polypharmacy 18
polyuria 123
portal circulation 9
positive efficacy 9
post-natal depression 160
post-traumatic stress disorder 148
postherpetic zoster pain 34
prazosin 132
prednisolone 97
pregnancy 21, 41, 88, 105–6, 137–8
preparations of local anaesthetics 37
prescribing law 186–8
prion 54
pro-drugs 6–7
procaine 36
product formulation 170
product packaging 170
prokaryotes 55, 58
prophylaxis 20, 61, 105
prostacyclin 86, 102
prostaglandins 33, 40–2, 87–8, 117
protease 65–6
protease inhibitors 65–6
protein binding 18
protein C 106
protein synthesis 58–60
protozoa 72–5
   amoeboflagellates 74
   apicomplexa 72–3
   definition 78
   flagellates 73–4
proviral DNA 65
pseudomembraneous colitis 60
psychological factors contributing to depression 152
psychosis 138, 157–60
   atypical antipsychotics 159
   definition 162
   drugs used in **158**
   side-effects 159–60
   typical antipsychotics 158–9
psychostimulants 160
PTSD *see* post-traumatic stress disorder

pulmonary embolism 105
pupillary constriction 44
pyrazinamide 63
pyrexia 75
pyridoxine 93

quinidine 107
quinine 73–4

ramipril 132
RCUK *see* Resuscitation Council
reboxitine 156
receptors 8
recombinant DNA technology 125
recreational drugs 22
recreational drugs *see* controlled drugs
referred pain 30
renal excretion 8–9
renal impairment 7, 41
reporting of drug errors 184–5
rescue remedies 118, 120
resistance 54, 58, 61, 73
resolution 85
respiratory depression 44, 46, 150
respiratory tract infection 75
resuscitation 20
Resuscitation Council 22
retroviruses 64–5
Review of Prescribing, Supply and Administration of
*   Medicines* 187
Reyes syndrome 41, 89
rheumatoid arthritis 12, 88, 173
ribonucleic acid 63–5
rifampicin 62–3
risk factors for asthma 117
risperidone 159
rivaroxaban 107
RNA *see* ribonucleic acid
rofecoxib 88
rosiglitazone 128
routes of administration **5**, 182
rubella 64

St John's wort 157
salbutamol 10, 19, 139
salmeterol 118
schizophrenia 134, 157–8, 160
Schwann cells 30
sedation 153, 160
selective serotonin re-uptake inhibitors 151, 154–6, *155*
selective toxicity 55
selegiline 134
sensation of pain 30–4
    body's analgesic system 33–4
    nerve impulse 30–1

neurones 30
    pain reception 31–3
sensory neurones 30
septicaemia 69
serotonin 8, 31, 33, 149, 154–6
    selective re-uptake inhibitors 154–6
sertraline 151
sexually transmitted diseases 64, 73
short-acting insulins 125
side-effects 170
    enoxaparin 105
    gentamycin 59
    histamines 90–1
    insulin 126
    penicillin 57
    psychosis 157–60
    quinine 74
    rifampicin 63
    steroids 90–1, **91**
    typical antipsychotics 159–60
    warfarin 106
smoking 121–2
    see also chronic obstructive pulmonary disease
sodium valproate 137–8, 142, 156–7
solubility 5
somatic pain 34
spinal anaesthesia 38
spinothalamic tracks 33, *34*
SSRIs *see* selective serotonin re-uptake inhibitors
Staphylococcus aureus 61
status asthmaticus 116
    see also asthma
status epilepticus 136
STDs *see* sexually transmitted diseases
steroids 89–91
    administration 90
    definition 96
    side-effects 90–1
'stocking-glove' distribution 35
stomatitis 92
streptokinase 109, 111
Stuart-Prower factor 105–7
subarachnoid space 38, *39*
subcutaneous routes 9
substantia gelatinosa 33
suicide 152, 156
sulfasalazine 92
sulfonylureas 127–8
sulpiride 159
Supply and Administration of Medicines under Group
*   Protocols* 186, 190
supply of drugs 186
surface area for absorption 4
swings of mood 156
synaptic vesicles 31

tachycardia 132, 136
tachypnoea 89
tardive dyskinesia 159
TCAs *see* tricyclic antidepressants
Temazepam 150
teratogenicity 138
terazosin 132
terbinafine 72
terfenadine 89
tetracyclines 58
theophylline 60, 119, 121
theory of planned behaviour 173
thiazide diuretics 130–1
thiazolidinediones 128
thrombocytopenia 105–6
thrombophlebitis 59
thromboplastin 102
thrombosis development 103
thromboxane 86, 102
thrush *see* candida
thyrotoxicosis 106
time of dosing 170
tinea 68
tinidazole 74
tinnitus 73, 89
Tinzaparin 105, 112
tissue pain 34
tolbutamide 127
topical allergies 22
topical anaesthesia 37
topoisomerase II 60
transcriptase inhibitors 65
transdermal patch 9, 45
transport systems 8
treatment of anaphylaxis 22
treatment with insulin 123–5
tri-fluoperazine 151, 163
trichomoniasis 74
tricyclic antidepressants 35, 151, 153–4
trigeminal neuralgia 30, 34–5
trimethoprim 55–6
true yeasts 68
tryptophan 156
tuberculosis 62–3
    isoniazid 62–3
    pyrazinamide 63
    rifampicin 63
tuberoinfundibular pathway 159
TXA$_2$ *see* thromboxane
Type A ADR 20

Type B ADR 20
type I/type II diabetes *see* diabetes mellitus
types of pain 34–6
    neuropathic pain 34–6
    nociceptive pain 34
typical antipsychotics 158–60
    mesolimbic pathway 158–9
    nigostriatal pathway 159
    side-effects of 159–60
    tuberoinfundibular pathway 159
tyramine 154

ulcerative colitis 94
underdosing 181–2
unionized compounds 7
unipolar depression 152
unwanted effects of local anaesthesia 39

Valium 180
valproate 137–8
vasoconstriction 37, 102
vasodilation 37, 39, 84, 102, 130
venlafaxine 156
venous thromboembolism 107
verapamil 132
vertigo *see* dizziness
vigabatrin 138
viral disease 63–4
    definition 76
    viral mechanisms 64
viral RNA 65
visceral pain 34
vitamin K 54, 57, 104, 106, 112
vomiting *see* nausea
VTE *see* venous thromboembolism

Wall, P. D. 33
warfarin 6, 21, 23–4, 42, 106–12
well-controlled asthma 139
WHO *see* World Health Organization
withdrawal symptoms 45, 138
World Health Organization 20, 39, 43, 61, 148

yeast-like fungi 69
yellow card system 20–2

zero efficacy 9–10
zidovudine 65
zona fasciculate 90
Zovirax 66

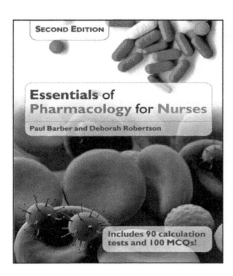

ESSENTIALS OF PHARMACOLOGY FOR NURSES 2/E

Paul Barber and Deborah Robertson

9780335245659 (Paperback)
May 2012

eBook also available

This popular book introduces pharmacology and calculations in a friendly, informative way and is now updated throughout with new topics and new coverage of more drugs and drug issues. The book focuses on the pharmacology knowledge needed at pre-registration level and does not assume previous knowledge of pharmacology, or a level of confidence with maths and drugs calculations.

Key features:

- Calculation sections containing 90 calculations to help perfect calculation skills
- 100 multiple choice questions to help the reader assess learning
- Patient scenarios from a range of different clinical settings, demonstrating pharmacology in clinical settings

www.openup.co.uk

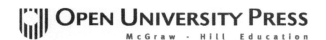

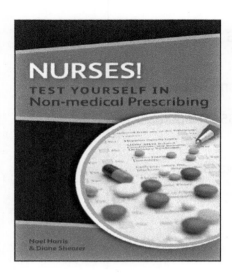

NURSES! TEST YOURSELF IN NON-MEDICAL PRESCRIBING

Noel Harris and Diane Shearer

9780335244997 (Paperback)
August 2012

eBook also available

Part of the '*Nurses! Test yourself in..*' series, this book covers the main topics from non-medical prescribing courses and modules that appear in the exam. This includes pharmacology and calculations as well as the legal, procedural and practical aspects of the prescribing role that are assessed on the course such as: drug safety, consultation skills, adverse drug reactions, concordance, using the BNF and special care groups such as children, pregnant women and mental health clients.

Key features:

- A range of question types, including True or False and Multiple Choice
- Questions based around mini-case scenarios for prescribing
- Provides a list of clearly explained answers to questions, so the book can be used as a 'teach and test' resource

www.openup.co.uk

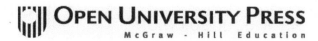

OPEN UNIVERSITY PRESS

McGraw - Hill Education